A Year by Design

A Year by Design

Kieran Ekeledo

CONTENTS

1	Choose Your Challenge	1
2	Celebrate Success	7
3	Learn From Losses	13
4	Know Yourself	20
5	Select Your Roles	33
6	Set Some Goals	42
7	Shortlist Your Top Ten Goals	58
8	Turning Goals to Reality	69
9	Generate £300,000 in Annual Turnover	82
10	Publish 33 Books	95
11	Make Memories With My Girlfriend	107
12	Celebrate Success with Family & Friends	118
13	Complete 72 Days of Champ Camp	130
14	Train Like a Fighter for 300 Days	143
15	Think Like a Champion for 300 Days	157
16	Level Up Like a Boss for 300 Days	171
17	Study Champions From The Bible	177

18 Feature 12 Times in Mainstream Media 184

19 Planners vs Trackers 191

20 Recommended Resources 212

1

Choose Your Challenge

Life is full of challenges, whether you're chasing your dreams or letting them fade into the background. But here's the truth: you get to choose your challenge.

Will you embrace the discipline it takes to pursue your goals, or will you settle for the regret of looking back on another year wondering what could've been? The fight isn't optional—it's part of life. The only choice is *how* you'll fight and *what* you'll fight for.

This book, *A Year by Design: A Step-by-Step Blueprint to My Best Life*, is about choosing the kind of fight that builds a life of purpose, growth, and success. It's a personal guide to how I, Kieran Ekeledo—The Boxing Life Coach—am making 2025 my best year yet by taking on challenges with clarity, intention, and strategy.

I'm not just setting goals; I'm stepping fully into the roles that matter most to me—Boss, Lover, Fighter, Champion, Man of God, Family Man, Boxing Life Coach, and Super Author. Each role reflects a part of who I am, and my top ten goals are the blueprint for fulfilling those roles.

The Power of Roles and Goals

When I started designing this year, I knew I needed more than vague ambitions. I needed clarity. I asked myself two key questions:

1. *Who do I need to become this year?*
2. *What do I need to achieve to step fully into those roles?*

This process wasn't just about listing accomplishments. It was about aligning my actions with my identity, my goals with my purpose. Each role is a lens through which I view my life, and each goal is a milestone on the journey to becoming the best version of myself.

My Roles for 2025

1. **Boss:** Running businesses with excellence, clarity, and ambition.
2. **Lover:** Building deeper intimacy and making weekly memories with my girlfriend.
3. **Fighter:** Training and thinking like a fighter, embodying discipline and resilience.
4. **Champion:** Living with the mindset of a winner, embracing success and learning from every loss.
5. **Man of God:** Studying biblical champions like Jesus, David, Moses, Samson, and Solomon to grow spiritually.
6. **Family Man:** Celebrating success and deepening connections with family and friends.
7. **Boxing Life Coach:** Inspiring others through my journey, teaching them to train like fighters and think like champions.
8. **Super Author:** Publishing 33 books to leave a legacy of knowledge, inspiration, and growth.

Each role reflects a different part of who I am and who I'm becoming. And each goal ties directly into one or more of these roles.

My Top 10 Goals for 2025

1. **Generate £300,000 in annual turnover.**
   This goal reflects my role as a Boss, proving that strategy, discipline, and leadership can turn vision into results.
2. **Publish 33 books.**
   As a Super Author, this is my way of leaving a lasting legacy, shar-

ing my knowledge, and inspiring others to take charge of their lives.

3. **Complete 72 days of Champ Camp.**
As a Fighter, Champ Camp is about pushing my physical and mental limits, building discipline, and sharpening my focus.

4. **Make weekly memories with my girlfriend.**
Love isn't just about words—it's about actions. This goal as a Lover is about prioritizing our connection and creating a foundation for a lifetime of shared joy.

5. **Celebrate success with family and friends.**
As a Family Man, I want to make time to share victories, both big and small, with the people who matter most.

6. **Train like a fighter for 300 days.**
This goal combines my roles as Fighter and Champion. It's about committing to the discipline of daily training to embody the mindset and physicality of a true fighter.

7. **Think like a champion for 300 days.**
Success isn't just about what you do—it's about how you think. This goal ties directly into my role as Champion, focusing on mindset, resilience, and mental toughness.

8. **Level up like a boss for 300 days.**
To lead effectively, I need to grow continuously. This goal is about investing in personal development, leadership skills, and strategic thinking.

9. **Study biblical champions.**
As a Man of God, studying figures like Jesus, David, Moses, Samson, and Solomon will help me grow spiritually and apply timeless wisdom to modern challenges.

10. **Feature in mainstream media 12 times.**
This goal as a Boxing Life Coach and Super Author is about expanding my reach, sharing my story, and inspiring others through TV, radio, and print features.

What's to Come in This Book

We're going to break down the process of designing your best year yet. This isn't just a guide to my journey—it's a toolkit for building your own.

Here's what you can expect:

1. Celebrate Success

Learn how to acknowledge and celebrate your wins, no matter how small. Success isn't just about the big moments—it's about the small steps along the way.

2. Learn from Losses

Every champion faces setbacks. This chapter will explore how to turn losses into lessons and use them as fuel for your next victory.

3. Know Yourself

Success starts with self-awareness. We'll dive into how to understand your strengths, weaknesses, and unique potential.

4. Select Your Roles

Who do you need to be this year? This chapter will guide you through defining the roles that align with your goals and values.

5. Set Some Goals

We'll explore how to set clear, actionable goals that reflect your vision for the year ahead.

6. Shortlist Your Top Ten Goals

Prioritisation is key. This chapter will help you narrow your focus to the ten goals that matter most.

7. Turn Goals Into Reality

It's not enough to dream big—you need a plan. This chapter will cover strategies for turning your goals into actionable steps.

8. A Step-by-Step Walkthrough of My Top Ten Goals

I'll take you behind the scenes of my personal goals for 2025, sharing how I plan to achieve each one.

9. Planners vs. Trackers

We'll discuss the difference between planning for success and tracking your progress, and how to use both effectively.

10. Resources for Success

Big dreams come with big risks. This chapter will help you assess risks, weigh rewards, and make bold but calculated decisions.

A Year Designed for Growth

Designing your best year isn't about perfection—it's about intention. It's about choosing your challenge, stepping into your roles, and committing to your goals with everything you've got.

As we move through this journey together, I encourage you to think about your own roles and goals. Who do you want to be this year? What do you want to achieve?

This is your time. Choose your challenge wisely. Let's make it count.

Choose Your Challenge

⊕	⊖
Chasing Dreams	Fading Dreams
Pain of Discipline	Pain of Regret
Setting Goals	Going with the flow
Clarity of purpose	Vague ambition
Strength	Weakness
Full Ownership	Victim of Circumstance

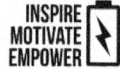

Fight For Success

2

Celebrate Success

When you're chasing big goals and dreaming of a better future, it's easy to forget to stop and acknowledge how far you've already come. But success, no matter how small, deserves celebration. Mike Tyson once said, *"Success breeds confidence, and confidence breeds success."* That quote resonates deeply with me because I've experienced firsthand how acknowledging your wins—big or small—fuels the momentum to achieve even greater things.

Celebrating success isn't just about patting yourself on the back; it's about building gratitude, focus, and self-belief. It's a moment to recognize that the hard work, sacrifices, and discipline are paying off. It's about saying to yourself: *I'm on the right path, and I've got what it takes to keep going.*

The Power of Celebration

In boxing, we celebrate victories in the ring. A knockout win isn't just a physical triumph; it's the culmination of months—sometimes years—of hard work. But in life, we often forget to raise our gloves and revel in the wins we achieve outside the ring. We get so focused on the next challenge, the next milestone, that we forget to pause and reflect on what's going well.

But here's the thing: celebrating success is fuel. It's a reminder of your resilience, your growth, and your ability to overcome. Whether you're closing a business deal, smashing a fitness goal, or simply being there for your loved ones, every victory deserves acknowledgment.

Reflecting on My Successes

As I look back on the past 12 months, I'm reminded of just how much there is to celebrate. The year wasn't perfect—no year ever is—but it was filled with moments that made me feel grateful, proud, and inspired to keep pushing forward.

Here are ten successes from the past year that I'm celebrating:

1. Giving My First Speech at The House of Lords

Stepping into the iconic halls of the House of Lords was surreal. As I stood before a room filled with influential figures, sharing my story and my mission, I felt a sense of purpose like never before. This wasn't just a personal victory—it was a moment that showed me how far I've come and how much further I can go.

2. Connecting and Collaborating with Football Legend Gianfranco Zola

Meeting Gianfranco Zola was more than just a highlight—it was a lesson in humility and greatness. Despite his legendary status, Zola's warmth and approachability left a lasting impression on me. Our collaboration reminded me that success doesn't have to come at the cost of kindness.

3. Securing My First Sponsor in KELF Civil Engineering

When I secured my first sponsor, KELF Civil Engineering, it wasn't just about the financial support—it was about validation. Someone believed in my vision enough to invest in it. That belief gave me even more confidence to keep pushing forward.

4. Making Over £10K Sales in a Month

Hitting five figures in sales in a single month was a testament to the power of focus and systems. This wasn't just a financial milestone—it was proof that the strategies I'd been refining were working.

5. Completing My First World Record: 120 Consecutive Rounds of Boxing Coaching

Breaking a world record was a physical and mental challenge like no other. Coaching 120 consecutive three-minute rounds required grit, endurance, and a deep connection with my "why." As I hit the final bell, I wasn't just exhausted—I was elated.

6. Celebrating Special Occasions with Family and Friends

Some of the most meaningful victories are the ones we share with the people we love. From birthdays to anniversaries, celebrating these moments with my family and friends reminded me of what truly matters.

7. Interviewing and Being Called an Inspiration by Legendary Boxing Coach Teddy Atlas

At the Anthony Joshua vs. Daniel Dubois weigh-in, I had the honor of interviewing the legendary Teddy Atlas. Hearing him call me an inspiration was a surreal moment—proof that my journey is resonating with others.

8. Finishing 30 Pull-Ups in One Set

Fitness has always been a cornerstone of my life, but completing 30 pull-ups in one set was a personal triumph. It reminded me that discipline and consistency yield results, no matter how long the journey.

9. Reading the Bible in One Year

This was more than just a spiritual goal—it was a commitment to growth, reflection, and connection with my faith. Reading the Bible in a year gave me new insights and strengthened my role as a Man of God.

10. Systemising My Personalised Boxing Life Coaching Experience

Creating a structured, scalable system for my boxing life coaching services was a game-changer. It allowed me to impact more lives while staying true to my mission of helping people train like fighters and think like champions.

Lessons from Champions

Celebrating success isn't just about listing accomplishments—it's about learning from them. Great fighters and champions know this. They take time to reflect on their victories, extracting lessons that will help them in the next round.

Sugar Ray Leonard: Confidence from Small Wins

Sugar Ray Leonard once said, *"Within our dreams and aspirations, we find our opportunities."* Leonard understood that each small win builds the confidence to chase bigger dreams.

Joe Louis: Consistency in Victory

Joe Louis, one of the greatest heavyweights of all time, celebrated every win as a stepping stone to the next. He knew that success isn't a destination—it's a journey of consistent effort and improvement.

Mike Tyson: Success Breeds Confidence

Mike Tyson's iconic quote, *"Success breeds confidence, and confidence breeds success,"* perfectly encapsulates why celebration matters. Each victory fuels the belief that you can achieve even more.

The Gratitude Factor

Celebrating success isn't just about you—it's about gratitude. Gratitude for the people who supported you, the lessons you've learned, and the opportunities you've been given.

For me, gratitude is woven into every success I celebrate. I'm grateful for my family, my team, my mentors, and my faith. I'm grateful for the challenges that pushed me to grow. And I'm grateful for the moments of joy, connection, and purpose that make the journey worthwhile.

The Call to Celebrate
Now it's your turn. Take 12 minutes to reflect on the past year. Write down 10 successes—big or small—that you're proud of.

Here are some prompts to get you started:

- What's one personal goal you've achieved this year?
- What's a professional milestone you're proud of?
- Who have you connected with or supported?
- What moments brought you joy, laughter, or gratitude?

Take your time with this exercise. Remember, every success matters.

Final Thoughts
Celebrating success isn't just an act of gratitude—it's an investment in your future. It's a reminder that you're capable, resilient, and deserving of greatness.

As we move forward in this book, we'll explore how to build on these successes, learn from challenges, and design a year that reflects the best version of yourself.

So take a moment to celebrate. Write down your wins. Relish the feeling of pride, gratitude, and possibility.

And remember: success breeds confidence, and confidence breeds success. Let's build that momentum together.

Celebrate Success

My Top Ten Wins for the past 12 months are:

1.
2.
3.
4.
5.
6.
7.
8.
9.
10.

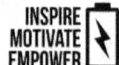

Fight For Success

3

Learn From Losses

In boxing, no one gets through their career undefeated. Even legends like Muhammad Ali, Sugar Ray Robinson, and Joe Louis experienced losses in the ring. But what set them apart was their ability to turn those losses into lessons. Ali famously said, *"Only a man who knows what it is like to be defeated can reach down to the bottom of his soul and come up with the extra ounce of power it takes to win when the match is even."*

This chapter isn't about wallowing in where we fell short—it's about acknowledging our missteps, extracting the lessons they offer, and using them as fuel to propel us forward. Because, just like in the ring, life's toughest rounds can teach us the most.

Looking back on 2024, I can see where I fell short. There were disappointments, unmet expectations, and goals that slipped through my fingers. But here's the truth: every one of those moments carried a lesson, and those lessons are shaping the game plan for my best year yet in 2025.

The Power of Losses

Losses hurt, whether they come from a fight in the ring, a missed business opportunity, or a personal setback. But they also offer clarity. They strip away excuses and force you to confront what's holding you back.

In 2024, I had my fair share of losses. Some were glaring, others subtle, but all of them taught me something. Here are ten areas where I fell short, along with the lessons they've taught me:

1. I Did Not Hit £10K a Month Consistently

While I had moments of financial success, I didn't sustain it month after month. Less than 50% of the time, I hit my target of £10K in monthly turnover.

Lesson: Consistency requires systems. I realized that my income goals can't rely on occasional big wins—they need a foundation of reliable processes and recurring revenue streams. In 2025, I'm focusing on creating automated systems that generate consistent income while leaving space for growth.

2. I Did Not Travel as Much as I'd Like

Traveling opens your mind and fuels your creativity. This past year, I let other priorities crowd out my opportunities to explore the world.

Lesson: Balance is key. While I was focused on building my businesses, I neglected the experiences that recharge my soul. For 2025, I'm committing to planning trips in advance and aligning them with my goals for growth and connection.

3. I Did Not Save as Much as I'd Like

Saving is about discipline and foresight. While I made strides in earning, I didn't prioritize setting aside enough for the future.

Lesson: Income without financial discipline leads to missed opportunities. In 2025, I'll be implementing a strict savings strategy, ensuring that every pound has a purpose.

4. I Did Not Invest Enough Time in Intimate Relationships

Relationships require nurturing, and this past year, I sometimes let my focus on work overshadow my personal connections.

Lesson: Love is a priority, not an afterthought. In 2025, I'm dedicating weekly time to make meaningful memories with my girlfriend, putting effort into growing our bond.

5. I Did Not Connect with the Woman of My Dreams

Building deep, meaningful relationships takes intentional effort, and this year, I fell short in pursuing the connection I envision.

Lesson: Clarity and commitment are vital. In 2025, I'm focused on clear communication, vulnerability, and prioritising love in all its forms.

6. I Was Not as Disciplined in My Training for Cardio and Conditioning

As someone who prides himself on training like a fighter, I let my conditioning slip in 2024.

Lesson: Your body is your foundation. In 2025, I'm recommitting to a structured training regimen that balances strength, cardio, and recovery.

7. I Did Not Give Any Keynote Talks Over £1,200+

Speaking engagements are a chance to inspire and expand my reach. While I gave meaningful talks, I didn't break through the financial ceiling I'd set for myself.

Lesson: Know your worth and communicate it effectively. In 2025, I'll be more intentional about pitching myself to organizations and negotiating fees that reflect the value I bring.

8. The Champions of Christ Community Did Not Grow to 10K+

I set an ambitious goal to grow the Champions of Christ community to over 10,000 members, but I fell short.

Lesson: Growth takes strategy and engagement. In 2025, I'm focusing on creating content, fostering connection, and leveraging social media to build this community.

9. I Only Completed the 10K Level Up Challenge 6/10 Times

The 10K Level Up Challenge is about pushing limits, and this year, I didn't fully rise to the occasion.

Lesson: Commitment means showing up, even when it's hard. In 2025, I'm doubling down on preparation and consistency to complete every challenge.

10. My Email List Is Under 1,000

Building a strong email list is essential for connecting with an audience, and I fell short of my target.

Lesson: Consistency and value create engagement. In 2025, I'll be focusing on providing valuable content and using creative strategies to grow my list.

Turning Pain Into Power

Losses sting. But they also carry the seeds of growth. Each setback I've faced in 2024 has given me clarity on where I need to improve and what I need to prioritise in 2025.

In boxing, every loss is an opportunity to adjust your strategy. After a tough fight, you and your coach watch the tape, analyze your performance, and figure out what went wrong. Did you drop your guard? Were you too aggressive? Did you underestimate your opponent?

Life is no different. Turning losses into lessons requires self-reflection, honesty, and a willingness to change.

Lessons From the Greats
Evander Holyfield: Hard Work and Faith

Holyfield once said, *"It's not the size of a man but the size of his heart that matters."* After his losses, Holyfield always came back stronger, using his faith and work ethic to fuel his comebacks.

Mike Tyson: Bouncing Back

Tyson's losses didn't define him—they refined him. He often spoke about the importance of learning from defeat, saying, *"I'm the greatest fighter in the history of the sport. Nobody had to endure pain the way I had to endure."*

Floyd Mayweather: The Power of Preparation

Mayweather's undefeated record isn't luck—it's the result of relentless preparation. He said, *"All work is easy work"*. Even setbacks in his personal life became lessons that sharpened his focus in the ring.

Lessons From My Journey

Every one of my losses in 2024 has taught me something. I've learned to focus on consistency over quick wins, to prioritise relationships, and to show up for myself and others with more discipline and intention.

Your Turn: Turning Losses Into Lessons

Now it's your turn. Take 12 minutes to reflect on the past year. Write down 7 areas where you fell short. Then, for each one, identify the lesson it taught you and how you can apply that lesson moving forward.

Here are some questions to help you get started:

- What goal did you miss, and why?
- What habit or mindset held you back?
- What positive lesson can you take from the experience?
- How can you use that lesson to improve in 2025?

Final Thoughts

Turning losses into lessons isn't easy, but it's one of the most powerful things you can do. Each setback is an opportunity to grow, to adjust, and to come back stronger.

As we move forward in this book, we'll explore how to build on these lessons, design a clear plan for the year ahead, and create a life that reflects the best version of yourself.

Losses are inevitable. Growth is a choice. Let's choose growth together.

Losses into Lessons

Loss	Lesson

Fight For Success

4

Know Yourself

If there's one thing I've learned in my journey as a fighter, coach, and human being, it's this: success starts with self-awareness. You can't achieve your goals—or even know what they are—if you don't understand who you are and what matters most to you. Knowing yourself is the foundation for everything else in life. It's your compass, your guide, and your anchor when the going gets tough.

In boxing, we say you fight the way you train. Similarly, in life, you move in the direction of your values. Your values are the principles that guide your decisions, shape your behavior, and ultimately define your success. They're the core of who you are.

For me, 2025 is all about living in alignment with my values. These values not only reflect who I am but also who I aspire to be as a Boss, Fighter, Champion, Man of God, Boxing Life Coach, Super Author, Lover, and Family Man.

But it wasn't always this way. There was a time when I drifted, moving aimlessly from one goal to the next without understanding why. Then life taught me a lesson: when you don't define your values, life defines them for you. And let me tell you, the world's version of success doesn't always align with what truly fulfills your soul.

Why Knowing Yourself Matters

When you know yourself, you gain clarity. You understand your purpose, priorities, and non-negotiables. This clarity helps you make better decisions, stay focused on what matters, and avoid distractions that pull you away from your goals.

Muhammad Ali once said, *"It's the repetition of affirmations that leads to belief. And once that belief becomes a deep conviction, things begin to happen."* Ali's quote isn't just about boxing—it's about life. Repeating the principles you live by, day after day, builds belief in who you are and what you stand for.

Think about fighters like Joe Louis or Sugar Ray Leonard. Their skill, grit, and determination weren't accidental. They were reflections of their inner values. Joe Louis had a quiet integrity that fueled his reign as heavyweight champion for over a decade. Sugar Ray Leonard's charisma and work ethic made him one of the most beloved fighters of all time. They knew who they were, and their values shone through in every punch, every fight, every triumph.

The same is true for us. When we know ourselves, we stop chasing empty victories and start living in alignment with what truly matters.

My 2025 Values and Why They Matter

For 2025, I've chosen 10 values to guide me. These aren't just words on a page—they're principles I strive to embody every day. They reflect my growth, my aspirations, and my commitment to becoming the best version of myself.

1. Faith

Faith is my foundation. It reminds me to trust in God's plan, even when the path isn't clear. My faith gives me strength, perspective, and hope. It's what keeps me grounded and focused on my purpose as a Man of God and Boxing Life Coach.

I remember a particularly challenging time early in my coaching career. I'd taken on a group of young fighters from a tough neighborhood. Many of them came from broken homes, and their struggles often spilled into the gym. One day, a boy named Aaron came to practice late, his face swollen from a fight he'd had at school. He was angry at the world, and that anger showed in the ring.

I didn't know what to say to him at first. But then I remembered my own struggles, the times I'd leaned on faith to find my way. I told Aaron about the importance of trusting in something bigger than ourselves, of believing that our pain has a purpose. Slowly, he began to listen. Today, Aaron is not only a better fighter but also a mentor to younger kids in the gym.

Faith doesn't just guide me—it helps me guide others.

2. Family

Family is my "why." It's the reason I push myself to grow, succeed, and create a legacy worth leaving behind. Celebrating special moments with my loved ones reminds me that success isn't just about personal achievements—it's about shared joy and connection.

One of my most cherished memories from 2024 was a family barbecue we hosted in the summer. The smell of grilled food filled the air, kids were laughing, and everyone was swapping stories around the table. For a moment, everything felt perfect.

That day reminded me of the power of presence. It's easy to get caught up in the hustle and forget to make time for the people who matter most. But those moments of connection fuel everything else we do.

3. Fitness

Fitness isn't just about looking good—it's about feeling strong, capable, and energized. As a Fighter, fitness is non-negotiable. It's a reflection of discipline, resilience, and commitment.

I'll never forget the first time I ran 10 kilometers without stopping. It was during a particularly grueling training camp. My legs felt like lead, and my lungs burned with every breath. But I kept going, one step at a time. When I finally crossed that imaginary finish line, the sense of accomplishment was overwhelming.

Fitness is more than physical—it's mental. It teaches you to push past limits, embrace discomfort, and discover what you're truly capable of.

4. Integrity

Integrity is about doing what's right, even when no one is watching. It's the cornerstone of trust, both in business and personal relationships. Living with integrity means staying true to my principles and being the kind of person others can count on.

In 2024, I had an opportunity to take on a lucrative sponsorship deal that didn't align with my values. It was tempting—I won't lie. But in the end, I turned it down. Why? Because integrity matters more than money. That decision reinforced my belief that success isn't just about what you gain—it's about how you gain it.

5. Hard Work & Dedication

Nothing worthwhile comes easy. Hard work and dedication are what separate the good from the great. As Mike Tyson said, *"Discipline is doing what you hate to do but doing it like you love it."* This value drives me to show up every day, no matter how I feel.

6. Discipline

Discipline is the bridge between goals and achievements. It's what keeps me consistent, focused, and moving forward, even when motivation fades. Discipline is the backbone of every successful fighter—and every successful person.

7. Resilience

Life will knock you down—it's inevitable. But resilience is what gets you back up. This value reminds me to embrace challenges, learn from setbacks, and keep fighting for what matters.

8. Confidence

Confidence isn't arrogance—it's belief in your abilities and your worth. It's what allows you to step into the ring, whether it's in business, relationships, or personal growth, and give it your all.

9. Kindness

Kindness is underrated but powerful. It's about treating others with respect, empathy, and generosity. As a Boxing Life Coach, kindness helps me connect with people and inspire them to become their best selves.

10. Vision

Vision is the ability to see what's possible, even when it's not yet visible. It's about dreaming big, setting bold goals, and staying focused on the bigger picture. Vision is what turns aspirations into reality.

Your Turn: Define Your Values

Now it's your turn. Take 12 minutes to reflect on what matters most to you. Write down your top 10 values and think about how they align with your goals, decisions, and actions.

To help you get started, here's a list of 50 values to consider:

1. Faith
2. Family
3. Fitness
4. Integrity
5. Hard Work & Dedication
6. Discipline
7. Resilience
8. Confidence
9. Kindness
10. Vision
11. Respect
12. Humility

13. Legacy
14. Creativity
15. Freedom
16. Growth
17. Gratitude
18. Leadership
19. Love
20. Perseverance
21. Accountability
22. Courage
23. Joy
24. Empathy
25. Adventure
26. Honesty
27. Passion
28. Purpose
29. Service
30. Patience
31. Loyalty
32. Innovation
33. Community
34. Compassion
35. Excellence
36. Balance
37. Wisdom
38. Generosity
39. Persistence
40. Spirituality
41. Self-Control
42. Determination
43. Optimism
44. Independence
45. Reliability

46. Authenticity
47. Fairness
48. Flexibility
49. Trust
50. Focus

Feel free to add your own values to the list.

Values

My Top Ten Values for the next 12 months are:

1.
2.
3.
4.
5.
6.
7.
8.
9.
10.

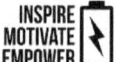

Fight For Success

Once you've chosen your top 10, it's time to complete a Success Scorecard.

Success Scorecard for *A Year by Design*

The **Success Scorecard** is a tool to help readers measure their progress and identify areas for growth as they work through the principles in *A Year by Design*. Each category aligns with a key aspect of designing and achieving your best life. Readers will score themselves from **1 to 10** in each category, with **1** representing "needs significant improvement" and **10** representing "fully mastered." The total score reflects their success rate as a percentage.

The 10 Categories

1. Goal Clarity

- Have you clearly defined your top goals for the year?
- Are they SMART (Specific, Measurable, Achievable, Relevant, Time-Bound)?

Score:

2. Daily Discipline

- Are you consistently taking action on your goals daily?
- Do you follow routines that align with your desired outcomes?

Score:

3. Resilience

- How well do you bounce back from setbacks or failures?
- Do you reframe challenges as opportunities to grow?

Score:

4. Mindset

- Are you actively cultivating a champion mindset through affirmations, visualization, and positive thinking?
- Do you practice gratitude regularly?

Score:

5. Health and Fitness

- Are you prioritizing physical health, including regular exercise, proper nutrition, and recovery?
- Are you training like a fighter or maintaining physical goals outlined in the book?

Score:

6. Relationships

- Are you investing time in building and maintaining meaningful connections with family, friends, and loved ones?
- Are you celebrating success with your nearest and dearest?

Score:

7. Faith and Spiritual Growth

- Are you deepening your spiritual practices, such as prayer, meditation, or studying biblical champions?
- Are you applying lessons of faith in your daily life?

Score:

8. Financial Growth and Management

- Are you on track with financial goals, like generating revenue, saving, or investing?
- Are you leveraging resources effectively to grow your wealth?

Score:

9. Legacy and Contribution

- Are you actively working to leave a positive impact on your community or industry?
- Are you mentoring, inspiring, or helping others achieve their goals?

Score:

10. Personal Growth and Learning

- Are you reading, learning, or acquiring new skills to improve yourself?
- Are you reflecting on lessons learned and implementing them in your life?

Score:

Scoring

1. Add up your scores for all 10 categories.
2. The total will give you your **Success Percentage**.

- **90-100%: Outstanding** – You're designing and living your best life! Keep the momentum going.
- **75-89%: Strong** – You're making great progress but can refine certain areas.
- **50-74%: Moderate** – You've laid the groundwork, but there's room for improvement.
- **Below 50%: Needs Attention** – You've got work to do, lets go back to fundamentals

Reflection and Next Steps

- Celebrate the areas where you scored highest—these are your strengths!
- Identify the categories where you scored lowest—these are opportunities for growth.
- Choose one low-scoring area to focus on improving this week.

This scorecard empowers readers to track their growth and remain accountable to their goals. By regularly reflecting and adjusting, success becomes inevitable.

Success Scorecard

The **Success Scorecard** is a tool to help readers measure their progress and identify areas for growth as they work through the principles in A Year by Design. Each category aligns with a **key aspect** of designing and achieving your best life. Readers will score themselves from 1 to 10 in each category, with 1 representing "needs significant improvement" and 10 representing "fully mastered." The total score reflects their success rate as a percentage.

- **90-100%: Outstanding** – You're designing and living your best life!
- **75-89%: Strong** – You're making great progress but can refine certain areas.
- **50-74%: Moderate** – You've laid the groundwork, but there's room for improvement.
- **Below 50%: Needs Attention** – You've got work to do, lets go back to fundamentals

Goal Clarity	/10
Daily Discipline	/10
Resilience	/10
Mindset	/10
Health and Fitness	/10
Relationships	/10
Faith and Spiritual Growth	/10
Financial Growth and Management	/10
Legacy and Contribution	/10
Personal Growth and Learning	/10
Total Score	/100

Fight For Success

Final Thoughts

Knowing yourself is the first step to designing your best year—and your best life. Your values are your foundation, your guide, and your source of strength.

As we move forward in this book, keep your values at the forefront. Let them guide your decisions, shape your actions, and inspire your journey.

Take 12 minutes today to define your values and score your current life. This simple exercise could change the way you see yourself—and the way you live your life.

When you know yourself, you find infinite opportunities for growth.

5

Select Your Roles

Who do you need to become to make this your best year yet? That's the question at the heart of this chapter. Every year is a chance to rewrite your story, but success doesn't happen by accident. It's the result of clarity, intention, and action—and that starts with defining the roles you need to play in your life.

Just like a fighter steps into the ring with a game plan, you need to step into the year with a clear understanding of who you are and the roles that matter most. These roles aren't just titles—they're reflections of your priorities, values, and goals. They're the foundation for the person you're becoming.

The Power of Roles

In boxing, every great fighter plays multiple roles. In the ring, they're warriors—relentless, disciplined, and focused. Outside the ring, they might be mentors, leaders, or family men. Muhammad Ali wasn't just "The Greatest" because of his talent in the ring. He was also an activist, a man of faith, and a voice for change.

The roles you choose define how you show up in the world. They guide your decisions, shape your behavior, and help you prioritize what matters most. When you're clear on your roles, you can align your actions with your purpose and create a life that's intentional and fulfilling.

My Roles for 2025

As I reflect on 2024 and look ahead to 2025, I've identified eight roles that are essential to who I am and who I'm becoming. Each role represents a part of my identity, my goals, and my vision for the future.

1. Boss

As a Boss, I'm committed to leading with vision, strategy, and integrity. This role is about stepping up as a leader in my businesses, making smart decisions, and creating opportunities for growth.

Being a Boss isn't just about financial success—it's about taking ownership of my life. It's about building something meaningful, staying disciplined, and setting an example for others.

2. Lover

Love is a priority, not an afterthought. As a Lover, I'm committed to nurturing my relationship with my girlfriend and building a foundation for a future together.

This role is deeply personal to me. One of my dreams is to have a wife and kids one day, and I know that building a strong relationship now is essential to creating that future. Love isn't just about grand gestures—it's about showing up consistently, being present, and creating moments of connection.

3. Fighter

As a Fighter, I'm committed to training like a champion, both physically and mentally. This role is about discipline, resilience, and pushing myself to be the best I can be.

Boxing has taught me countless lessons about life. It's shown me the power of hard work, the importance of staying focused, and the resilience it takes to keep going when things get tough. Training isn't just about fitness—it's a metaphor for life.

4. Champion

Being a Champion is about mindset. It's about approaching life with confidence, focus, and a relentless drive to succeed.

In 2024, I learned the importance of thinking like a champion. Whether it was breaking a world record for consecutive rounds of boxing coaching or hitting personal milestones in my career, every success started with the belief that I could achieve it.

5. Man of God

Faith is at the core of who I am. As a Man of God, I'm committed to growing spiritually, studying biblical champions, and living in alignment with my faith.

In 2024, I read the Bible in one year—a goal that deepened my understanding of God's word and strengthened my relationship with Him. For 2025, I'm focusing on studying figures like Jesus, David, Moses, Samson, and Solomon, drawing lessons from their lives to guide my own.

6. Family Man

Family is everything. As a Family Man, I'm committed to creating meaningful connections, celebrating successes, and supporting the people I love.

One of my favorite moments from 2024 was hosting a family gathering where we laughed, shared stories, and simply enjoyed each other's company. These moments remind me that success means nothing if you can't share it with the people who matter most.

7. Boxing Life Coach

As a Boxing Life Coach, my mission is to inspire, motivate, and empower others to achieve their goals in fitness, business, and life.

This role is one of the most fulfilling parts of my journey. Helping others train like fighters and think like champions isn't just about boxing—it's about transforming lives.

8. Super Author

Writing is one of the most powerful ways to share knowledge, inspire change, and leave a legacy. As a Super Author, I'm committed to publishing 33 books in 2025—a goal that reflects my passion for storytelling and personal growth.

The Long-Term Vision

These roles aren't just about 2025—they're about the life I'm building. I see myself as a husband, father, leader, and mentor. I want to create a legacy that inspires others to live with purpose, integrity, and passion.

Selecting these roles is a way of aligning my daily actions with my long-term vision. It's about becoming the person I'm meant to be and helping others do the same.

Your Turn: Define Your Roles

Now it's your turn. Take 12 minutes to reflect on the roles that matter most to you. Who do you need to be to make this your best year yet?

Here's a list of 100 roles to consider:

Family Roles

1. Parent
2. Partner
3. Husband
4. Wife
5. Father
6. Mother
7. Son
8. Daughter
9. Sibling
10. Grandparent
11. Uncle
12. Aunt

13. Cousin
14. Guardian
15. Caregiver

Personal Development Roles

16. Student
17. Teacher
18. Mentor
19. Mentee
20. Dreamer
21. Visionary
22. Thinker
23. Innovator
24. Writer
25. Creator
26. Listener
27. Friend
28. Advocate

Professional Roles

29. Boss
30. Entrepreneur
31. Leader
32. Manager
33. Strategist
34. Builder
35. Planner
36. Problem-Solver
37. Designer
38. Marketer
39. Investor

40. Speaker
41. Trainer
42. Influencer
43. Networker
44. Healer
45. Consultant
46. Analyst

Health & Fitness Roles

47. Fighter
48. Athlete
49. Coach
50. Trainer
51. Adventurer
52. Competitor
53. Wellness Advocate
54. Nutritionist

Spiritual Roles

55. Man of God
56. Woman of Faith
57. Believer
58. Servant Leader
59. Disciple
60. Seeker

Community Roles

61. Volunteer
62. Activist
63. Community Leader

64. Philanthropist
65. Caregiver
66. Connector

Creative Roles

67. Super Author
68. Artist
69. Musician
70. Designer
71. Filmmaker
72. Storyteller

Adventure Roles

73. Explorer
74. Traveler
75. Pioneer
76. Risk-Taker

Relationship Roles

77. Lover
78. Friend
79. Confidant
80. Supporter

Leadership Roles

81. Captain
82. Coach
83. Guide
84. Facilitator

Personal Growth Roles

85. Challenger
86. Builder
87. Planner
88. Achiever

Legacy Roles

89. Historian
90. Archivist
91. Elder
92. Custodian

Other Roles

93. Organizer
94. Innovator
95. Mediator
96. Peacemaker
97. Helper
98. Motivator
99. Protector
100. Advocate

Feel free to add your own roles to the list. Once you've chosen your top 8, write a brief description of why each one matters to you.

Final Thoughts

Selecting your roles is one of the most powerful steps you can take toward designing your best year. These roles define who you are, what you prioritize, and how you show up in the world.

Take 12 minutes today to reflect on your roles. Write them down, commit to them, and let them guide your actions in 2025.

When you're clear on who you are, there's no limit to what you can achieve.

Role Rolodex
My Top Eight Roles for the next 12 months are:

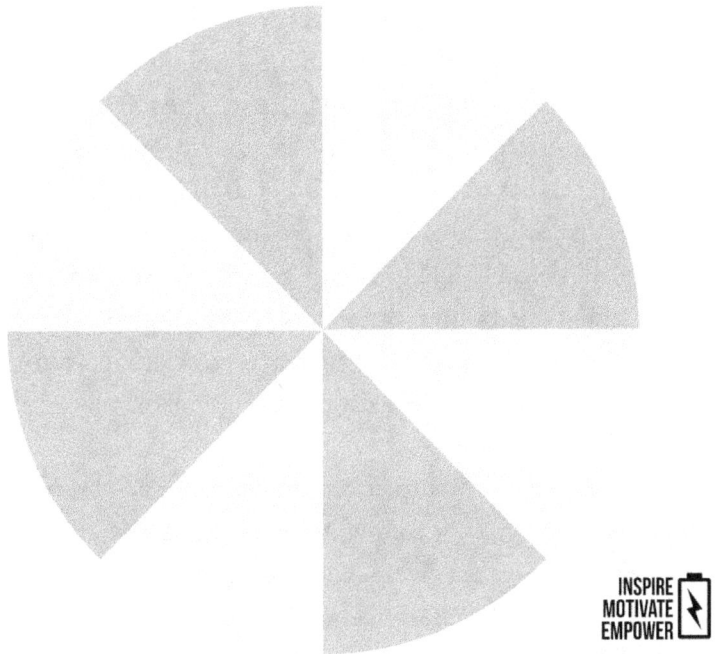

Fight For Success

6

Set Some Goals

When I step into the gym, gloves on, sweat beading down my face, I'm reminded that every fight—whether in the ring or in life—is won or lost by how well you prepare. The same principle applies to designing your year. If you want to emerge victorious, you need a game plan. And that starts with setting clear, powerful goals.

Goal-setting might sound like old news. We've all heard about SMART goals before—making them. Specific, Measurable, Achievable, Relevant, and Time-bound. But theory is one thing; practice is another. This chapter is about putting it into action, aligning your goals with your roles, and making them so inspiring and doable that you can't wait to get started.

I've chosen eight roles to focus on in 2025: Boss, Lover, Fighter, Champion, Man of God, Family Man, Boxing Life Coach, and Super Author. Each role reflects who I want to be, how I want to show up in the world, and what I want to accomplish. By setting goals for each role, I'm ensuring that every aspect of my life gets the attention it deserves.

As we go through this, I'll share how to set goals that align with your identity, fit the SMART criteria, and drive you forward every day. And at the end, I'll challenge you to do the same. Let's get started.

The Power of Setting SMART Goals

Before diving into each role, let's revisit what makes a goal "SMART":

- **Specific:** Clearly define what you want to achieve. Avoid vague language.
- **Measurable:** You must be able to track progress and know when you've hit the target.
- **Achievable:** The goal should stretch you, but still be realistic.
- **Relevant:** It should matter to you and align with your values and purpose.
- **Time-bound:** Give yourself a deadline or timeline for completion.

For example, saying "I want to get fitter" is vague. A SMART version might be: "I will run a 10K in under 50 minutes by June 30th." You know exactly what you're aiming for, by when, and you can measure your performance.

Setting Goals for My 8 Roles
1. Boss

As a Boss, I'm the leader of my entrepreneurial pursuits and business ventures. This role demands vision, strategy, and a willingness to adapt. It's about financial growth, strategic partnerships, and setting the tone for a thriving enterprise.

Goals:

1. **Increase Monthly Turnover:**

    - *Specific:* Generate £300,000 in annual turnover by December 31, 2025.
    - *Why:* To ensure financial stability and invest in team growth.
    - *How:* Break it down into quarterly targets, secure at least 3 high-value clients per quarter, and review financials monthly.

2. **Launch a Flagship Product or Service:**

    ◦ *Specific:* Launch a new premium coaching program by February 1, 2025, aimed at helping business owners lose weight and fight for success, in and out the ring. Apply boxing principles to their business strategy.
    ◦ *Why:* To diversify revenue streams and showcase my unique approach.
    ◦ *How:* Partner with boxing gyms, health clubs, boxing promoters, coaches and health and wellness professionals.

3. **Grow influence and impact within the boxing industry:**

    ◦ *Specific:* Implement a new community management system (like Patreon or Skool) by February 28, 2025, to streamline content and exclusive access to behind the scenes interviews..
    ◦ *Why:* Better communications leads to consistent quality and happier clients.
    ◦ *How:* Train the team on Skool and Patreon,, run a pilot in February, measure outcomes in March.

2. Lover

As a Lover, this role is about nurturing my relationship. It's not just date nights; it's about genuine connection, communication, and building a future together.

Goals:

1. **Weekly Quality Time:**

   - *Specific:* Make memories weekly with my girlfriend—no phones, just conversation and connection—every Sunday evening.
   - *Why:* To strengthen our bond and create shared memories.
   - *How:* Book restaurants in advance, surprise her with a new activity each month, and track consistency on a calendar.

2. **Quarterly Adventures:**

   - *Specific:* Take one weekend trip every quarter (4 trips in 2025) to explore new places together.
   - *Why:* Shared experiences deepen intimacy and keep things fresh.
   - *How:* Discuss destinations in January, April, July, October; plan budgets and itineraries together.

3. **Shared Goals Check-In:**

   - *Specific:* Sit down every month to discuss our personal and shared goals for 2025.
   - *Why:* Aligning our visions and supporting each other's growth.
   - *How:* Put it in the calendar—30 minutes on the last Saturday of each month. Review successes, challenges, and dreams.

3. Fighter

As a Fighter, I embody discipline, courage, and resilience. It's about pushing my physical and mental limits, drawing strength from hardship, and always getting back up.

Goals:

1. **72 Days of Champ Camp Completion:**

   - *Specific:* Complete all 72 days of Champ Camp by December 31, 2025.
   - *Why:* To sharpen my fitness, discipline, and tenacity.
   - *How:* Schedule the camp days, mark them off as done, and track improvements in stamina and strength.

2. **300 Training Days a Year:**

   - *Specific:* Train like a fighter for 300 days, which means planned workouts, recovery sessions, and skill drills.
   - *Why:* Consistency builds conditioning and mental toughness.
   - *How:* Mark training days on a calendar, review monthly, and never miss two days in a row.

3. **Running Milestone:**

   - *Specific:* Increase my running endurance—go from 5km to 8km a day by June 30, 2025.
   - *Why:* To push my limits and improve ring fitness.
   - *How:* Add one extra 1km every two months, focusing on technique and breathing.

4. Champion

Being a Champion isn't just about winning fights—it's a mindset of unwavering self-belief, mental resilience, and a hunger for growth. It's about thinking like a champion every day.

Goals:

1. **300 Champion Mindset Days:**

    - *Specific:* Spend 5 minutes daily on mental training—visualisation, affirmations, or reading inspiring quotes—300 times in 2025.
    - *Why:* To reinforce confidence, focus, and resilience.
    - *How:* Set a reminder for mornings, track the habit in a journal.

2. **Quarterly Goal Reflection:**

    - *Specific:* Every quarter, review my biggest wins, losses, and lessons learned.
    - *Why:* Champions learn from every outcome.
    - *How:* Block out one hour at the end of March, June, September, and December for reflection.

3. **Interview a Champion:**

    - *Specific:* Interview at least one successful champion—could be a boxer, entrepreneur, or community leader—by August 31, 2025.
    - *Why:* To learn their mindset strategies and apply them to my life.
    - *How:* Reach out via email, Instagram or LinkedIn, prepare questions, record the interview, and take notes.

5. Man of God

As a Man of God, I lean into faith for guidance, wisdom, and purpose. Studying biblical champions and strengthening my spiritual life keeps me grounded and aligned with my calling.

Goals:

1. **Study 5 Biblical Champions:**

   - *Specific:* By November 30, 2025, complete in-depth studies of Jesus, David, Moses, Samson, and Solomon.
   - *Why:* Their stories offer lessons on faith, leadership, courage, and wisdom.
   - *How:* Dedicate 30 minutes twice a week to reading scripture and commentary. Take notes and reflect on how their stories apply to my life.

2. **Faith Journal:**

   - *Specific:* Write a 5-minute faith reflection daily for 200 days in 2025.
   - *Why:* To keep my relationship with God central and learn from spiritual insights.
   - *How:* Journal right after morning prayer or before bed, track consistency.

3. **Service Project:**

   - *Specific:* Volunteer for at least one faith-based community project by September 30, 2025.
   - *Why:* Faith without works is empty. Serving others is living the gospel.
   - *How:* Find a local church initiative, sign up early, dedicate a weekend to making a difference.

6. Family Man

A Family Man invests in relationships that matter most—celebrating successes, supporting each other through struggles, and building a legacy of love and connection.

Goals:

1. **Monthly Family Dinners:**

    - *Specific:* Host or attend a family dinner at least once a month throughout 2025.
    - *Why:* To strengthen family bonds and create shared memories.
    - *How:* Put it on the calendar—last Friday of each month, rotate who hosts.

2. **A Family Celebration:**

    - *Specific:* Organise a family gathering to celebrate key achievements by July 31, 2025.
    - *Why:* To share in the joy of wins—like hitting my business target or finishing Champ Camp—and appreciate our support system.
    - *How:* Book a venue or prepare a home-cooked feast, send invitations a month in advance.

3. **Legacy Conversations:**

    - *Specific:* Have 4 in-depth conversations with family elders about their stories, advice, and dreams (one per quarter in 2025).
    - *Why:* Understanding family history and wisdom enriches identity and perspective.
    - *How:* Plan calls or visits, record notes, and reflect on lessons learned.

7. Boxing Life Coach
Boxing Life Coach Goals:

1. **Launch a Signature Coaching Program: Key Results Club**

    - *Specific:* Develop and launch a 12-week online coaching program by February 1, 2025, blending boxing principles with personal development strategies. There will also be a 12 month option for those who want to commit to a bigger transformation with exclusive access to sparring classes and boxing shows.
    - *Why:* To reach a broader audience, provide structured guidance, and help participants train like fighters and think like champions. Add entertainment and games aspect to your coaching to your program.
    - *How:* Outline modules in January, film and edit content in February and March, run a beta test in March 22-23, and go live on May 1.
    - *Measure of Success:* Achieve at least 3 Elite Champions, 7 Diamond Lions and 12 Gold Tigers, 27 Iron Tigers sign-ups in the first month and gather positive feedback to refine the program.

2. **Feature in Mainstream Media 12 Times**

    - *Specific:* Secure 12 appearances in mainstream media—TV segments, movie documentaries, radio interviews, or print articles—by December 31, 2025.
    - *Why:* To expand reach, build credibility, and inspire more people with the Boxing Life Coach philosophy.

- *How:* Pitch to at least 2 media outlets monthly, showcase client success stories, and highlight unique coaching methods.
- *Measure of Success:* Total of 12 confirmed features by year's end, with at least one high-profile outlet included.

3. **Client Transformation Spotlights**

    - *Specific:* Identify and highlight 3 client transformation stories by October 31, 2025—document their journey from start to finish, including before-and-after progress and personal testimonials.
    - *Why:* To demonstrate the tangible impact of my coaching methods and inspire potential clients.
    - *How:* Track participants' progress over a 3-6 month period, interview them, and compile their stories into short videos or written case studies.
    - *Measure of Success:* Publish these 3 transformation stories on my website and share across social media, aiming for increased engagement and new client inquiries.

4. **Grow Coaching Community by 20%**

    - *Specific:* Increase membership in my coaching community (online group or subscription service) by 20% by September 30, 2025.
    - *Why:* A larger, more engaged community creates a supportive environment, enhances learning experiences, and amplifies word-of-mouth referrals.
    - *How:* Offer monthly Q&A sessions, consistently post valuable training and mindset content twice a week, and introduce a referral incentive program.
    - *Measure of Success:* Track membership numbers monthly and celebrate reaching the 20% growth milestone with a special event or bonus seminar.

8. Super Author

As a Super Author, writing 33 books in a year is a bold target. It's about leaving a legacy of wisdom, motivating others, and sharing my experiences to help them navigate their own paths.

Goals:

1. **33 Books Published:**

   - *Specific:* Publish 33 books by my birthday, May 27th, 2025 (about 31 books to go. April 29th 2025 will be a big release day, with other books and workbooks being published around that date)
   - *Why:* To create a body of work that inspires others, cements my legacy, and proves what's possible with vision & discipline.
   - *How:* Plan and prepare daily, set a word count target, schedule editing and formatting processes, and release books consistently.

2. **Diverse Formats:**

   - *Specific:* Experiment with different formats—at least 3 audiobooks, 2 workbooks, and 1 graphic guide by December 31, 2025.
   - *Why:* Reach different audiences, keep creativity flowing.
   - *How:* Outsource audiobook narration, collaborate with a designer for the graphic guide, plan the workbook layout early.

3. **Reader Engagement:**

    ◦ *Specific:* Host a live virtual book reading or Q&A each quarter in 2025.
    ◦ *Why:* Interacting with readers builds community, garners feedback, and increases impact.
    ◦ *How:* Schedule events every 3 months, promote in advance, record sessions for later viewing.

The Importance of SMART Goals in Each Role

Notice how each goal is SMART. For example, in the Boss role, "Increase monthly turnover" is specific (£300,000 annual), measurable (track monthly revenue), achievable (based on previous performance and plans), relevant (it supports my business vision), and time-bound (by December 31, 2025).

When goals are SMART, they're not just dreams. They become targets you can aim for, measure progress against, and know exactly when you've achieved them.

Personal Stories and Inspirations

I've mentioned before how boxing legends integrated their goals into daily routines. Take Mike Tyson, who said, "Discipline is doing what you hate to do but doing it like you love it." He set clear training goals and stuck to them religiously, knowing they would lead to victory in the ring.

Or consider entrepreneurs like Muhammad Yunus (Nobel Peace Prize winner for microfinance): he set specific targets for how many small loans he'd provide to impoverished communities. Those goals, well-defined and monitored, changed the lives of millions.

In my own journey, when I decided to become a Super Author, I didn't just say, "I'll write a lot." I set a target of 33 books. That forced me to structure my writing time, stay disciplined, and treat writing like training. Each day of writing became like another round in the ring—focused, purposeful, and pushing my limits.

30 Potential Fitness Goals for Inspiration

Maybe one of your roles is Fighter, Athlete, or Champion, and you're looking for fitness-related goals. Here are 30 potential SMART fitness goals, mostly focused on running, triathlons, boxing, and calisthenics:

1. Run a 5K in under 25 minutes by June.
2. Complete a 10K race without walking by May.
3. Increase weekly running mileage from 10 miles to 20 miles by September.
4. Improve 1-mile personal best by 30 seconds by October.
5. Run a half-marathon under 2 hours by November.
6. Complete a full marathon by December 31.
7. Place in the top 50% of a local 5K race by August.
8. Finish a sprint triathlon by July.
9. Complete an Olympic-distance triathlon by September.
10. Improve swimming freestyle 100m time by 10 seconds within 3 months.
11. Bike 100 miles in a week by October.
12. Increase cycling speed average by 2 mph over 30 miles by June.
13. Master a full triathlon (Ironman 70.3) by year-end.
14. Join a boxing gym and attend 2 classes per week for 3 months.
15. Complete 3 rounds of sparring without gassing out by April.
16. Learn and perfect 5 new boxing combos by March.
17. Improve jump rope speed to 150 skips/min by May.
18. Achieve 50 push-ups in a row by July.
19. Perform 10 unbroken pull-ups by September.
20. Do a muscle-up within 6 months.
21. Hold a 3-minute plank by April.

22. Improve burpee count from 20 to 30 in a set by June.
23. Master 10 one-legged squats (pistols) by November.
24. Complete a calisthenics circuit (push-ups, pull-ups, squats) daily for 30 days.
25. Increase handstand hold time to 30 seconds by August.
26. Complete 5 rounds of a boxing HIIT circuit without rest by October.
27. Improve punch output to 100 punches/min for 2 straight minutes by May.
28. Land 50 double-unders in a row with a jump rope by July.
29. Learn to shadowbox with good form for 3 rounds by February.
30. Improve recovery by measuring resting heart rate and decreasing it by 5 bpm by year-end.

Each of these can be adapted to SMART criteria by adding specific deadlines, measurable targets, and reasons why they matter to you.

Your Turn: Make It Personal

You've seen how I'm setting goals across my eight roles. You've read a list of possible fitness goals. Now it's your turn. Goals become transformative when they're personal, aligned with your values, and genuinely excite you.

Take 12 minutes right now. Write down your top roles—maybe not eight, maybe you have six or nine—and then for each role, set 3-5 SMART goals. Remember: specific, measurable, achievable, relevant, and time-bound.

- Don't just say, "I want to be healthier." Say, "I will run a 10K in under 55 minutes by June 30, and I'll do it because I want more energy to play with my kids."
- Don't just say, "I want a better relationship." Say, "I will schedule a date night every Friday at 7 pm with my partner, and

surprise them with a new activity once a month, because I value our connection and long-term happiness."

Align these goals with your chosen roles. If you're a Family Man, maybe it's about monthly dinners, quarterly family trips, or family fitness challenges. If you're a Boss, it might be revenue targets, product launches, or team development milestones.

The Boxing Life Coach Mindset

As your Boxing Life Coach, I want you to remember that setting these goals is like crafting your fight plan. We're not just randomly punching—every goal is a planned jab, a strategic hook, a well-timed uppercut. Each one brings you closer to that year-end victory, where you raise your arms in triumph, knowing you gave it your all.

Great fighters like Floyd Mayweather talked about careful planning and precise execution. Business icons like Steve Jobs or Oprah Winfrey stressed clarity and intention in their pursuits. Relationship gurus emphasize showing up consistently and meaningfully. Faith leaders remind us that what we strive for should align with higher principles. Every champion in every field achieves greatness through well-defined goals and daily effort.

Wrapping Up

Goal-setting isn't a one-time event. Revisit these goals monthly, track your progress, and don't be afraid to adjust if life throws you a curveball. Remember the 12 key principles of success—faith, vision, teamwork, focus, hard work & dedication, discipline, the will to win, resilience, confidence, respect, humility, and legacy—and let them guide you as you pursue your goals.

This chapter has given you a framework and examples to work with. Now it's time to step into the ring with your pen and paper, commit to a plan, and start swinging.

Call to Action

Invest 12 minutes now. Take your roles and write down 3-5 SMART goals for each. Make them personal, challenging, and aligned with who you want to be. The world's greatest champions don't just dream—they write down their targets and attack them with relentless passion.

Set the timer, grab a notebook, and turn your roles into a roadmap of achievement. You've got this, champ.

Roles & Goals

The Role is:

The Goals are:

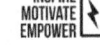

Fight For Success

7

Shortlist Your Top Ten Goals

Stepping into the ring—whether literally, as a fighter, or metaphorically, in life—requires clarity, focus, and conviction. You can have big dreams, an inspiring vision, and even a strong plan, but until you pinpoint the exact targets you're aiming for, you're still swinging blind.

In the previous chapters, we've explored who we need to be (our roles), what we value, and how to set goals that align with our identity. Now, it's time to narrow it all down. Out of all the possibilities, which goals will take centre stage in your year ahead?

This chapter is about selecting your top ten goals—those that best represent the roles you've chosen and the year you're designing. I'm going to walk you through my own selection process, show you how I'm aligning each goal with a particular role, and demonstrate how having a concise, powerful set of targets can energise your entire year.

By the end, you'll see how I've chosen one key goal for each of my eight roles, added an extra goal for my major role, and picked one more from the remaining possibilities to round out my top ten. As always, my process is just an example—adjust it to fit your own journey. Then, I'll encourage you to invest just 12 minutes to do the same and set yourself up for success.

From Many to a Mighty Few

I've got plenty of ambitions for 2025. Over the past few chapters, I've brainstormed goals for each of my roles: Boss, Lover, Fighter, Champion, Man of God, Family Man, Boxing Life Coach, and Super

Author. Now the challenge is to pick one standout goal for each role—something that captures the essence of what I'm striving for.

But I'm also going to choose an extra goal from my major role (the role I want to emphasise above all others this year) and then pick one final goal from the leftover options, giving me a total of ten goals.

Why limit myself to ten? There's nothing magical about the number, but ten is manageable. It's enough to cover every area I care about, without scattering my focus too thin. Ten goals feel like a championship fight card—enough to keep me engaged and challenged, but not so many that I lose track.

My Eight Roles

Let's recap the roles I've committed to focusing on in 2025:

1. **Boss**: The entrepreneurial leader in me, guiding my business ventures, making strategic decisions, and pushing for growth.
2. **Lover**: The partner who prioritises connection, love, and building a future with my significant other.
3. **Fighter**: The one who trains with discipline, embraces discomfort, and strives for physical and mental resilience.
4. **Champion**: The mindset master, nurturing confidence, resilience, and a winning attitude in everything I do.
5. **Man of God**: The spiritual seeker, grounding my actions in faith, wisdom, and divine purpose.
6. **Family Man**: The person who invests in family bonds, celebrates togetherness, and values legacy and love at home.
7. **Boxing Life Coach**: The mentor who uses boxing principles to inspire others, teach discipline, and transform lives.
8. **Super Author**: The creator of words, sharing knowledge, stories, and insights through the written page to leave a lasting legacy.

Selecting the Top Goals

Now, I'll pick my major role. Next, let's choose one core goal from each role. After that, select an additional goal from the major role. Finally, I'll add one last goal from the remaining pool to complete the top ten.

1. Boss: Generate £300,000 in Annual Turnover

- **Goal:** Generate £300,000 in annual turnover by December 31, 2025.
- **Why This Goal?** As a Boss, I want my business efforts to reflect strategic growth and financial stability. This figure challenges me to push beyond my comfort zone, find better clients, streamline operations, and invest wisely.
- **Personal Note:** I've always admired entrepreneurs who turned their passions into profitable, sustainable ventures. This goal ensures I'm not just talking about success, but building it—pound by pound.

2. Lover: Make Memories Weekly with My Girlfriend

- **Goal:** Create one special memory each week with my girlfriend—no phones, no distractions, just quality time.
- **Why This Goal?** Love thrives on consistency. This goal keeps our relationship vibrant, reminding me that the sweetest moments aren't grand gestures but steady, heartfelt presence.
- **Personal Note:** I think of legendary champions like Muhammad Ali, who, despite global fame, valued personal connections. If the greatest could appreciate the power of love and loyalty, so can I.

3. Fighter: Complete 72 Days of Champ Camp

- **Goal:** Finish all 72 days of Champ Camp by October 31, 2025.
- **Why This Goal?** Champ Camp is about forging discipline through structured training. Completing it ensures my body and mind are battle-ready, strengthening my will and resilience.
- **Personal Note:** Fighters like Mike Tyson dominated because they embraced brutal training. If I embrace the grind like they did, I'll become stronger in body and spirit.

4. Champion: Think Like a Champion for 300 Days

- **Goal:** Dedicate at least 5 minutes each day, for 300 days this year, to mindset work—visualisation, affirmations, or reading inspiring quotes.
- **Why This Goal?** Winning starts in the mind. By committing to daily mental conditioning, I'm ensuring my attitude remains confident, focused, and driven.
- **Personal Note:** Sugar Ray Leonard said, "Within our dreams and aspirations we find our opportunities." Thinking like a champion creates the mental environment where opportunities flourish.

5. Man of God: Study Biblical Champions (Jesus, David, Moses, Samson, Solomon)

- **Goal:** Complete an in-depth study of these five biblical figures by November 30, 2025, reflecting on their qualities and lessons.
- **Why This Goal?** Their stories offer spiritual guidance, leadership lessons, and moral insights I can apply to my life and work.

- **Personal Note:** Faith has always been my anchor. Understanding these champions' journeys helps me grow closer to God and more aligned with my purpose.

6. Family Man: Celebrate Success with Family and Friends

- **Goal:** Host or attend a family/friends gathering at least once a month, using it as an opportunity to celebrate wins—both big and small.
- **Why This Goal?** Success means more when it's shared. By making celebration a monthly habit, I keep loved ones at the heart of my victories.
- **Personal Note:** When I remember great champions like Evander Holyfield and Muhammad Ali, I recall how they valued family and community. Connecting with family keeps my feet on the ground and my heart open.

7. Boxing Life Coach: Feature in Mainstream Media 12 Times

- **Goal:** Appear in mainstream media (TV, movies, online, radio, or print) 12 times by December 31, 2025.
- **Why This Goal?** To expand my reach, inspire a wider audience, and show others how boxing principles can transform their lives.
- **Personal Note:** Exposure builds credibility. If Teddy Atlas, an iconic boxing trainer, can influence millions through media appearances, I can follow in that tradition to help more people discover their inner champion.

8. Super Author: Publish 33 Books

- **Goal:** Publish 33 books by December 31, 2025.

- **Why This Goal?** Writing is my legacy-building tool. These books will share knowledge, motivate readers, and demonstrate what's possible when you apply the 12 key principles of success to life..
- **Personal Note:** Think of authors who left indelible marks—Maya Angelou, Paulo Coelho. They wrote with purpose. Publishing 33 books is ambitious, but it proves that a Super Author can turn relentless creativity into a library of inspiration.

Choosing My Major Role and Its Extra Goal

I've got eight goals—one from each role. Now I need to pick a major role, one I'll emphasise even more, and add a second goal from that area. Which role calls out to me most for extra focus this year?

As I consider the impact I want to have, the Boxing Life Coach role stands out. It's my platform for helping others harness boxing's power to transform their lives. I want to dig deeper into this role, offering more structured programs and building a thriving community.

Extra Goal for My Major Role (Boss):

- **Goal:** Level Up Like a Boss for 300 days
- **Why This Goal?** Beyond just generating revenue and media appearances, I want to grow the business to the point where I can grow a team and change more people's lives. It's a way to create lasting impact and show I'm not just talking—I'm walking, empowering, and guiding others to success.
- **Personal Note:** I think about the way Freddie Roach shaped champions in his Wild Card Gym. He didn't just coach; he created systems and structures. He trained other coaches and built a team. The man is a true inspiration. .

That gives me 9 goals total: 8 from each role plus one extra from my major role, Boxing Life Coach.

One Final Goal from the Remaining Pool

SHORTLIST YOUR TOP TEN GOALS

Now, I have a range of goals that didn't make the initial cut. I want to pick one more that adds flavor, challenge, and another dimension to my year. Since I've already picked goals from each role, this final goal can come from any leftover ideas. I've got plenty: train like a fighter for 300 days, develop a 12 week online program, or maybe add another dimension to my growth.

From my previous brainstorming, I recall "Train like a fighter for 300 days" as an appealing goal. It complements my Fighter role (which already has Champ Camp) but pushes me further towards daily discipline.

Final Goal: Train Like a Fighter for 300 Days

- **Goal:** Engage in structured training sessions for 300 days this year, focusing on conditioning, technique, and mental toughness.
- **Why This Goal?** Completing Champ Camp is a milestone, but training consistently beyond those 72 days ensures I maintain peak condition and mental resilience year-round.
- **Personal Note:** Consistency is king. Mike Tyson didn't become Iron Mike by training sporadically—he did it daily, consistently, relentlessly. I can channel that spirit to become my own version of iron-willed.

Now I have my top 10 goals:

1. **Boss (Main Goal):** Generate £300,000 in annual turnover.
2. **Lover:** Make weekly memories with my girlfriend.
3. **Fighter:** Complete 72 days of Champ Camp.
4. **Champion:** Think like a champion for 300 days.
5. **Man of God:** Study biblical champions (Jesus, David, Moses, Samson, Solomon).
6. **Family Man:** Celebrate success with family and friends.
7. **Boxing Life Coach:** Feature in mainstream media 12 times.

8. **Super Author:** Publish 33 books.
9. **Boss (Extra Goal):** Level Up like a boss for 300 days
10. **Fighter (From the Leftover Pool):** Train like a fighter for 300 days.

Why These Ten Goals?

Together, these ten goals cover every corner of my life. From spiritual growth (Man of God) to business success (Boss), from personal relationships (Lover, Family Man) to public impact (Boxing Life Coach, Super Author), and from mental conditioning (Champion) to physical prowess (Fighter), these goals ensure that I'm not leaving any role behind.

They also challenge me in different ways: mental resilience, creative output, financial performance, relationship-building, and physical endurance. This diversity ensures I'm evolving as a whole person, not just excelling in one area at the expense of the others.

As legendary champion Manny Pacquiao said, "If you work hard in training, the fight is easy." By selecting a balanced set of goals, I'm ensuring that each "fight"—each area of my life—gets proper training. Each goal serves as a round in the grand bout of my year, keeping me sharp, engaged, and always moving forward.

Learning from Champions

Think of great champions like Muhammad Ali, who declared he was "The Greatest" long before the world agreed. He had clear, bold goals and pursued them relentlessly, adapting his training, mindset, and strategy as needed. Or consider entrepreneurs like Sara Blakely of Spanx, who started with a clear goal—reshape the women's undergarment market—and turned it into a billion-dollar company. She didn't do it by accident; she set targets and innovated tirelessly.

In love, consider athletes like Roger Federer, who balanced a thriving family life with his tennis career. He set personal boundaries and routines to ensure he could be present for his loved ones, even while chasing

Grand Slam titles. That balance required clear personal and professional goals working in harmony.

In every domain, the champions who stand out had a vision, picked their battles, and set targets that guided their decisions. That's what this top ten list is about—giving yourself a roadmap to follow, a standard to hold yourself against, and a reason to wake up excited each morning.

Your Turn: Invest 12 Minutes

Now it's your time to step into the ring. You don't have to follow my roles or my goals. Instead, think about what matters most to you. Take the roles you've defined in previous chapters—maybe you have fewer or more than eight—and select goals that truly resonate.

Action Step: Spend 12 minutes right now finalizing your top ten goals. Here's how:

1. **List Your Roles:** Identify the roles that define you. Maybe you have 5, 7, or even 10 roles.
2. **One Goal Per Role:** Pick one powerful goal that captures the essence of each role.
3. **Choose a Major Role:** Select your main role for the year and add an extra goal for it.
4. **Add One More Goal:** From your leftover ideas, pick one final goal to complete your top ten.
5. **Review for Balance:** Ensure these goals cover different areas of your life so you're growing holistically.

Set a timer for 12 minutes and do it now. Don't overthink—trust your instincts. By the time the bell dings, you'll have a lean, focused set of targets that guide your year and keep you moving forward.

Final Thoughts

Shortlisting your top ten goals is like tightening your gloves before a big match. You've done the warm-up, the shadowboxing, and the mental prep. Now you're ready to step into the ring with clear, tangible targets. These goals will keep you disciplined, direct your efforts, and ignite the drive to push through challenges.

As the Boxing Life Coach, I encourage you to remember the principles we've learned: faith, vision, teamwork, focus, hard work & dedication, discipline, the will to win, resilience, confidence, respect, humility, and legacy. Let these principles guide you as you chase your dreams, forging a path to a year of purpose and achievement.

The bell has rung. It's time to fight for your future, one smartly chosen goal at a time.

Top Ten Goals

My Top Ten Goals for the next 12 months are:

1.
2.
3.
4.
5.
6.
7.
8.
9.
10.

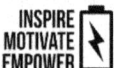

Fight For Success

8

Turning Goals to Reality

We've identified our goals, chosen our roles, and anchored ourselves in the values that matter most. We're painting the picture of our best year. But how do we take these dreams from ideas on paper to results in our hands? It's one thing to say, "I want to lose 10kg in the next three months," and it's another thing to see the scale confirm that you've done it. Turning goals into reality requires a **strategic approach**—one that moves beyond wishful thinking and into the realm of action.

In boxing, it's not just about knowing you want to win—you need a game plan. You study your opponent, understand what shots to throw, when to move, and how to handle unexpected blows. The same applies to life goals. Without a plan, you're shadowboxing against thin air. With a plan, you're more like Floyd Mayweather Jr —calculating, strategic, and prepared to execute when the bell rings.

This chapter dives into a five-part framework that I use to bring goals from imagination into reality: Gratitude, Outcome, Activities, Leverage, and Score. Think of these steps as your corner team, each one offering something you need to **dominate the ring of life**.

The GOALS Framework: Gratitude, Outcome, Activities, Leverage, Score

G.O.A.L.S Framework
Turning Goals to Reality

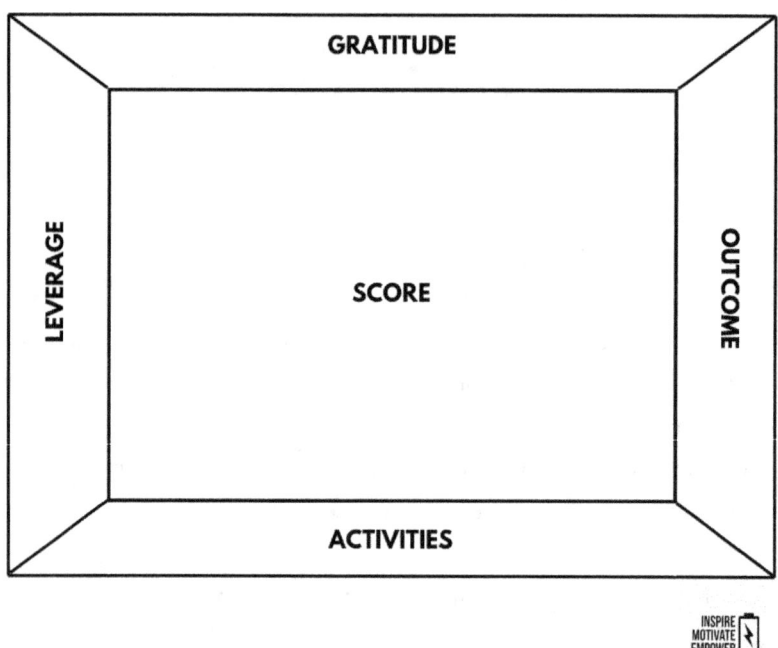

Fight For Success

Before we dive into each step, let's lay out what we're working with:

Gratitude: Start from a place of appreciation. Recognise what you already have, what's already working, and use that foundation to build something even greater. Gratitude gives you perspective and humility, keeping you grounded as you strive for more.

Outcome: This is where you define exactly what you want to achieve. Make it clear, measurable, and meaningful. Your outcome is the vision that guides your actions. It's the destination on the map, ensuring you know where you're headed and why you're going there.

Activities: Goals don't achieve themselves—you need to reverse-engineer them into daily, weekly, and monthly tasks. Identify the habits, routines, and milestones that form the path from where you are to where you want to be.

Leverage: No champion fights alone. Who can help you along the journey? Who has the knowledge, experience, or support that can expedite your progress? Surrounding yourself with the right people and resources can shorten your learning curve and keep you accountable.

Score: Finally, you must track your progress. Measure your lead and lag indicators, celebrate wins, and make adjustments when you're off track. Scoring keeps you honest and ensures you're actually moving closer to your goal, not just spinning your wheels.

Gratitude: The Foundation of Growth

Before you chase new heights, take a moment to appreciate where you stand. Gratitude is powerful. It reminds you that while you're aiming for more, you're not coming from nothing. You've got strengths, opportunities, and achievements that got you this far.

I remember a time in my boxing coaching career when I felt frustrated. I'd set a goal to expand my client base by 30% in a quarter, but progress felt slow. Instead of wallowing in disappointment, I took a step back and considered what I was grateful for: the clients I already had who trusted me with their fitness journeys, the small improvements I saw in them week after week, the fact that I was doing work I loved. Suddenly, my perspective shifted. Gratitude doesn't mean settling—it means acknowledging your blessings and using them as a springboard.

If you want more, first take stock of what you have. If your goal is to lose 10kg, start by appreciating your current health, the ability to move, the gym you have access to, or the supportive friends and family cheering you on. Gratitude grounds you, ensuring you approach your goals from a place of abundance rather than lack.

Action Step: List 10 things you're grateful for that relate to your goal. If losing 10kg is your aim, maybe you're grateful for the friend who joins you on morning runs, the local park with a running trail, or the nutritionist who gave you great meal prep tips. This exercise fuels positivity and motivation.

As a great champion, Joe Louis, once emphasized through his actions (not as many quotes survive as with Ali or Tyson), humility and recognition of what you have is key. He never forgot his roots and that kept him balanced through highs and lows. Gratitude does the same for you—it keeps you balanced as you reach higher.

Outcome: Defining Your Target with Precision

Now that you've got gratitude fueling your engine, it's time to pinpoint exactly where you're headed. Ambiguous goals lead to ambiguous results. This is why we stress making goals SMART: Specific, Measurable, Achievable, Relevant, and Time-bound.

- **Specific:** Instead of "I want to lose weight," say "I want to lose 10kg."
- **Measurable:** You know exactly how much weight you want to lose.
- **Achievable:** 10kg in 3 months might be challenging, but still within reason for most people, depending on their starting point.
- **Relevant:** Does this goal matter to you? Maybe it improves your health, energy, and confidence.
- **Time-bound:** You've given yourself three months.

For me, one of my big goals is to publish 33 books in a year(well actually whilst I'm 33 so I have until 27th May 2025). Sounds massive, right? But I break it down: 33 books, 5 months, that's about 7 books every month. I know my reasons: I want to share knowledge, inspire people, and create a lasting legacy as a Super Author. By having a clear outcome, I stay focused. The same applies to losing 10kg—it's not just about looking better, it's about feeling healthier, having more energy, and being able to keep up with your kids.

Action Step: Write down your outcome. For the 10kg goal, write: "I will lose 10kg in the next 3 months by following a structured nutrition and exercise plan." Then write why it matters. Why do you want this? Maybe it's to improve your health markers, your confidence, or your performance in the gym. Create a list of reasons why this goal is a must. What happens if you don't achieve this goal? Read these reasons daily—it's your source of motivation.

Sugar Ray Leonard said, "Within our dreams and aspirations we find our opportunities." Defining your outcome clearly allows you to see the opportunities hidden within your goal, giving you the clarity to seize them.

Activities: The Roadmap to Achievement

A goal without a plan is just a wish. This is where many people stumble—they know what they want, but they don't map out the path to get there. Activities turn your outcome into a step-by-step roadmap.

If losing 10kg is your target, what activities will get you there? Maybe:

- Meal prepping every Sunday for the week ahead.
- Doing cardio three times a week for 30 minutes.
- Strength training twice a week to build muscle and boost metabolism.
- Tracking daily calorie intake using an app.
- Weighing yourself once a week to monitor progress.

These are your checkpoints, the habits and routines that will bridge the gap between "I want to lose 10kg" and "I've lost 10kg." Think of them as the jabs, hooks, and uppercuts you throw to win the fight. Each activity is a move that gets you closer to victory.

In my own journey, when I aimed to generate £300,000 in annual turnover, I knew I needed actionable steps: identifying new clients, creating automated marketing funnels, delivering consistent quality content, and reviewing financials weekly. Without these action steps, my revenue goal would remain a number on a page.

Action Step: For each goal, list 3-5 activities that, if done consistently, will lead to success. Schedule these activities into your calendar.

If it's weight loss, when and where do you exercise? What day do you meal prep? Make it tangible and real.

Muhammad Ali used to say, "I run on the road before dancing under the lights." He understood that the activities you do in the shadows—early morning runs, late-night gym sessions—make the victory under the bright lights possible.

Leverage: Harnessing People, Knowledge, and Accountability

Champions don't rise alone. Even solo sports like boxing have coaches, mentors, sparring partners, and nutritionists behind the scenes. Leverage is about tapping into resources that amplify your efforts.

If you're aiming to lose 10kg, who can help? A personal trainer can give you exercise routines. A friend with cooking skills can teach you quick, healthy meal recipes. An online community focused on weight loss can offer support and accountability. By surrounding yourself with the right people, resources, and knowledge, you shorten the learning curve and stay motivated.

When I wanted to become a Boxing Life Coach who could genuinely transform lives, I sought out mentors—people who'd trained champions, coaches who understood the mental game. I attended seminars, read books, and joined mastermind groups. This wasn't cheating; it was smart. I leveraged other people's experience so I could improve faster.

Action Step: Identify at least 3 forms of leverage for your goal. For losing 10kg:

1. A friend who's into fitness to join your morning workouts.
2. A meal prep service or nutrition guide to simplify healthy eating.
3. A fitness tracker or online community for accountability.

Floyd Mayweather, undefeated as a boxer, always credited his father and uncle for their training and guidance. He understood the power of leverage—absorbing knowledge from those who've walked the path before you.

Score: Measuring Progress and Making Adjustments

Imagine a boxing match without judges, no scorecards, no idea who's winning. It'd be chaos. Similarly, in goal achievement, you need to measure your progress. This is where scoring comes in.

Set Key Performance Indicators (KPIs) for your journey. For weight loss, your lag measure is the scale weight—after three months, did you lose 10kg? But rely only on lag measures and you won't know if you're on track until it's too late. Instead, also track lead measures—the daily or weekly activities that predict success. Maybe your lead measures are the number of workouts per week, or the number of meals eaten at home instead of a restaurant.

You might weigh yourself weekly and note if you're losing around 0.8-1kg a week (which would keep you on track for 10kg in 12 weeks). If you're off track after week two, you can adjust. That's the beauty of scoring—you catch mistakes early.

When I aim to publish 33 books in a year, I don't wait until December to see if I'm on track. I measure how many chapters I write per week, how many hours I dedicate to editing, and how many pages I draft daily. These are my lead measures that predict whether I'll hit the final number.

Action Step: For each goal, decide how you'll measure progress. Is it weight on the scale, income in your bank account, number of pages written, or hours spent practicing a skill? Determine both lead and lag indicators. Check in weekly to note progress and make necessary adjustments.

Champions like Evander Holyfield reviewed fight tapes, assessed their strengths and weaknesses, and adapted accordingly. Treat your journey like a fighter studying performance. Score your progress and use it to become better week by week.

G.O.A.L.S Framework

Goal & Role: _____

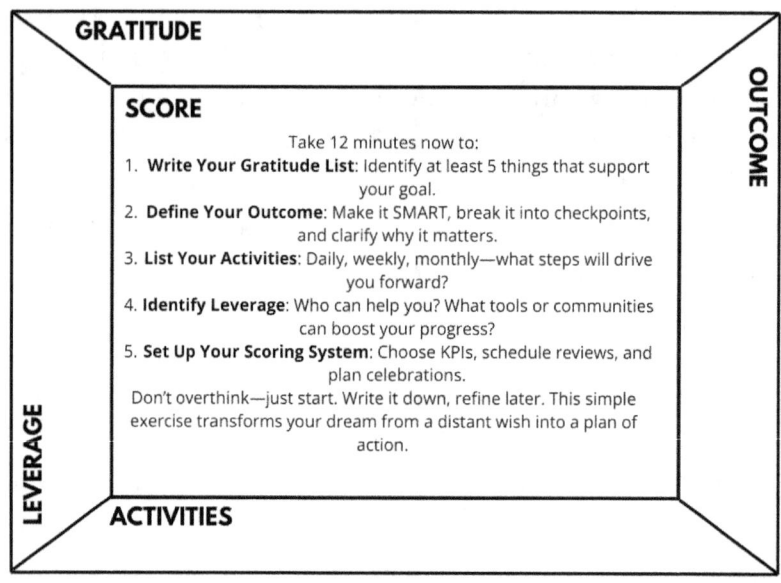

SCORE

Take 12 minutes now to:
1. **Write Your Gratitude List**: Identify at least 5 things that support your goal.
2. **Define Your Outcome**: Make it SMART, break it into checkpoints, and clarify why it matters.
3. **List Your Activities**: Daily, weekly, monthly—what steps will drive you forward?
4. **Identify Leverage**: Who can help you? What tools or communities can boost your progress?
5. **Set Up Your Scoring System**: Choose KPIs, schedule reviews, and plan celebrations.

Don't overthink—just start. Write it down, refine later. This simple exercise transforms your dream from a distant wish into a plan of action.

Fight For Success

A Practical Example: Losing 10kg in 3 Months Using GOALS
Let's walk through the entire process with the weight loss example:
Gratitude:

- Grateful for a supportive spouse who encourages my fitness journey.
- Grateful for having access to a gym nearby.
- Grateful for good health and the physical ability to exercise.
- Grateful for a friend who's a nutritionist and can offer advice.
- Grateful for technology that can track my calories and workouts easily.

By starting here, you embrace a positive mindset. Instead of feeling like you're starting from scratch, you realize you have advantages. This fuels motivation and resilience.

Outcome:

- I will lose 10kg in 3 months, going from 80kg to 70kg by March 31st.
- Why it matters: I want to feel more energetic, improve my health, fit into my favorite clothes again, and boost my confidence. This goal aligns with my vision of living a more active, fulfilled life.

Activities:

- Exercise: Cardio (running or cycling) 3x a week for 30 minutes, Strength training 2x a week.
- Nutrition: Meal prep on Sundays, follow a calorie-controlled diet, limit processed sugars.
- Tracking: Weigh-in every Monday morning, track food intake daily with an app.
- Sleep: Aim for 7-8 hours of sleep per night to support recovery and metabolism.

Each activity builds toward the outcome. Without these concrete steps, the goal remains intangible.

Leverage:

- Accountability partner: A friend who checks in with you each week on your progress.
- Expert knowledge: Consultation with a nutritionist or personal trainer for a meal plan and workout routine.
- Community: Join an online fitness group for tips, motivation, and success stories.

- Technology: Use a fitness tracker (Fitbit, Apple Watch) to monitor your daily steps, heart rate, and calorie burn, follow online or personalised training apps.

With these resources, you're not going it alone. You've got a support system to push you forward.

Score:

- Lead KPIs: Number of workouts completed per week (aim for 5), number of home-cooked meals per week (aim for at least 18 out of 21), daily calorie intake (~500 calories less than maintenance).
- Lag KPI: Weekly weigh-in results. You should see roughly 0.8-1kg loss per week to stay on track for 10kg in 12 weeks.
- Adjust: If after 2 weeks you're not losing at least 1.5-2kg total, you may need to tweak your diet or increase workout intensity.
- Celebrate: For each 3kg lost, treat yourself to a new workout outfit or a spa day. When you hit 10kg, plan a celebratory event with friends or buy that item you've been eyeing to reward your hard work.

By following this GOALS framework, you transform a vague dream ("I want to lose weight") into a concrete plan with steps, support, and measurement. This is how you turn goals into reality.

Embracing the Principles of Success

The GOALS framework isn't just for weight loss—it applies to any target, whether it's generating £300,000 in turnover, publishing 33 books, or featuring in mainstream media 12 times. The principles remain the same. Each step aligns with the 12 key principles of success we've been touching on: Faith (believe you can achieve it), Vision (define your outcome clearly), Teamwork (leverage your resources), Hard Work & Dedication (execute the activities), Discipline (stay consistent), The Will to Win (don't give up), Resilience (bounce back when off track), Confidence (act as if you belong), Respect (show manners and good courtesy), Humility (never stop learning) and Legacy(make a difference that inspires, motivate and empowers).

When you integrate these principles into the GOALS framework, you're not just hitting targets—you're becoming the person capable of sustained success. You're living like a champion in all areas of life: business, boxing, love, faith, and family.

The Bigger Picture

Remember, this process is part of "A Year By Design." You're not living a random year—you're designing it, crafting it, shaping it into the masterpiece of your life. Goals are the pillars of that masterpiece, and the GOALS framework is your blueprint.

As a Boxing Life Coach, I've seen countless clients come in with big dreams but no plan. Those who succeed are the ones who break their dreams into tangible steps and stick to the process, adjusting as needed. They understand that turning goals into reality is less about sudden breakthroughs and more about consistent execution over time.

The world's greatest champions in business, boxing, and beyond have followed similar formulas. Whether it's an entrepreneur building a startup into a global powerhouse or a fighter training every morning before sunrise, the pattern is clear. They know what they want, they create a plan, they use resources, they measure progress, and they adapt as necessary.

A Call to Action

Now it's your turn. Don't just read about this framework—apply it. Take one of your top 10 goals for the year and run it through the GOALS framework:

1. **Gratitude:** Write down at least 5 things you're grateful for that will help you achieve this goal.
2. **Outcome:** Clearly define your goal, make it SMART, and write down why it matters to you. Break the goal down into 3-5 checkpoints.

3. **Activities:** Identify the daily, weekly, and monthly habits you need to adopt in each phase. Schedule them.
4. **Leverage:** Find at least 3 forms of leverage—people, resources, communities—that can help you.
5. **Score:** Determine your lead and lag KPIs. Decide how often you'll measure progress and how you'll celebrate wins.

Spend 12 minutes doing this exercise right now. The clarity you gain will be worth far more than the time invested.

Final Thoughts

Turning goals into reality is not magic—it's a method. It's about starting with gratitude, defining a clear outcome, breaking it down into activities, seeking leverage from others, and keeping score of your progress. This systematic approach transforms you from a dreamer into a doer, from someone who talks about goals into someone who achieves them.

As legendary champion Manny Pacquiao once said, "If you work hard in training, the fight is easy." Apply the same logic to your goals: work hard in planning and execution, and the results will come more naturally.

You have the blueprint. You have the principles. Now, it's time to fight the good fight—one punch, one step, one day at a time—until your goals stand as undeniable, tangible reality.

G.O.A.L.S Framework

Goal & Role: _____

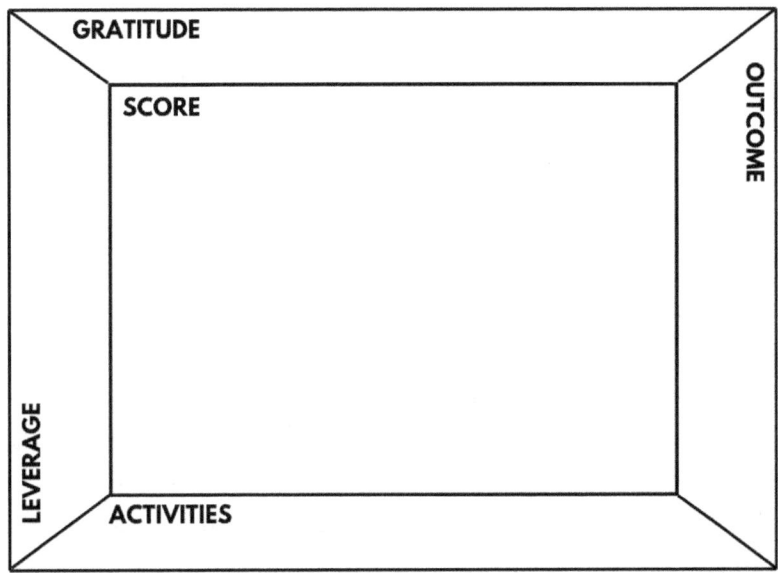

Fight For Success

9

Generate £300,000 in Annual Turnover

When I first stepped into the boxing gym, I didn't know how far the sport would take me. I knew I wanted to be stronger, fitter, maybe learn to throw a decent left hook. But I never imagined that one day I'd be using the principles I learned in that ring—discipline, focus, resilience—to build a thriving, purpose-driven business.

Today, I see the world of entrepreneurship much like a boxing match. Each financial goal is a title fight, and each round demands strategy, skill, and heart. In 2025, one of my major goals is to generate £300,000 in annual turnover. Why £300,000? Because it's a milestone that pushes me beyond my comfort zone and positions me for even greater impact. It's not just about the money—it's about what the money represents: freedom, opportunity, the ability to give back, and the chance to show others what's possible.

In this chapter, I'll apply the GOALS framework—Gratitude, Outcome, Activities, Leverage, and Score—to break down exactly how I plan to achieve this figure. The process I'm about to share is the same one I want you to embrace for your own goals, financial or otherwise. If you approach your ambition like a fighter prepares for a championship bout, you'll develop the resilience, confidence, and relentless spirit needed to win.

Gratitude: Embrace the Foundation of Your Strength

Before we chase new heights, let's ground ourselves in what we already have. Gratitude is like the ring floor under your feet—it's the stable surface from which you launch every punch, every move. Without gratitude, goals become desperate grasps for more. With gratitude, they become expressions of growth and contribution.

I'm grateful for so many things that position me for success in generating £300,000 this year:

1. **Past Experience in Revenue Generation:** I've generated over £300,000 turnover multiple times for other companies within 12 months. This proves I can deliver significant results when I apply myself fully. My best year was during the pandemic when I generated over £550,000 for Premier Global NASM, the leading fitness education company in the UK at the time.

2. **Previous Wins in My Own Business:** I've made over £10,000 in a single month before for my business. That's tangible evidence of my capabilities and my market's willingness to invest in what I offer.

3. **A Network of High-Performing Entrepreneurs:** I'm friends with multiple entrepreneurs who surpass £300,000+ turnover. Their guidance, insight, and support provide a roadmap and inspiration.

4. **Inspirational Examples of Personal Development Titans:** Legends like Tony Robbins, James Clear, David Goggins, Bedros Keullian, Alex Hormozi, Matt Fiddes and Joe Wicks have built empires from their expertise. They've proven that personal development and coaching can be extremely lucrative and impactful.

5. **Direct Coaching from Successful Entrepreneurs:** I've been coached by people who've already crossed the £300,000 mark—Tony Robbins, Mac Attram, Jordan Belfort, Samuel

Leeds, Paul O'Mahony. Their strategies and lessons are part of my toolkit.

Gratitude reminds me that I'm not starting from zero. I have experience, connections, and role models to draw upon. This isn't a blind leap—it's a calculated advance, supported by past success and existing strength.

Outcome: Clarify the Target and Why It Matters

Every great fighter enters the ring with a clear outcome: to win. But "win" isn't enough; we need specifics. In boxing, that might mean winning by knockout before the final round. In business, it means defining the exact revenue figure, timeframe, and strategy.

My Outcome:

- **SMART Goal:** I will generate £300,000+ in annual turnover by December 31, 2025.
- **Revenue Streams:**

  1. **Book Sales:** Aim for 15,000 sales at £20 each. That alone could bring £300,000 when fully realised, but I'll use multiple streams to diversify.
  2. **Key Results Club Subscriptions:**

     - Iron Eagles: 2,500 subscribers at £12 per month.
     - Gold Tigers: 250 clients at £500 a month for 3 months.
     - Diamond Lions: 25 clients at £1,200 a month for 12 months.
     - Elite Champions: 12 clients at £25,000 a time payment for 12 months.

3. **Affiliate Sales:** Partner with Amazon, Hyperice, PunchTrunk, KELF—these could add extra revenue from commissions.
4. **Sponsorships:** 10 sponsors at £30,000 each would be huge, even if hitting that might be ambitious.
5. **Google Ads / YouTube Revenue:** With a target of 100 million views across YouTube and my personal blog, significant ad revenue could stack up.
6. **Unique Partnerships:** Collaborations or joint ventures with other entrepreneurs or brands.

Checkpoints:

1. £30k earned: This proves viability early on.
2. £30k in a single month: Shows scalability and system efficiency.
3. £100k cumulative: A psychological milestone proving I'm on the right track.
4. £150k cumulative: Halfway mark—time to accelerate or pivot strategy.
5. £300k total by year-end: The final victory.

My Why: Money is never just money. For me, £300,000+ means:

- **Lifestyle & Security:** Top-notch healthcare, investing in my education, paying bills with ease, and enjoying stress-free living.
- **Family & Love:** Treating my family and friends, traveling to beautiful places like Marbella, Accra, Tokyo, Australia, Saudi Arabia. Supporting loved ones, saving for an engagement ring, wedding, and even property.
- **Professional Investment:** Funding the production of my 33 books, expanding Champ Camp, and scaling my business systems.

- **Legacy & Impact:** Inspiring others by sharing my journey, proving what's possible, giving back to the Church, mental health charities, helping my community.
- **Freedom & Options:** The confidence that comes with financial abundance, giving me the ability to help my sisters, nieces, nephews, and parents. Upgrading my lifestyle (fixing my teeth, buying a van for business) and celebrating successes (Tudor watch, Vision Pro sunglasses).

When I visualize that £300,000, I see more than numbers. I see my loved ones smiling, I see personal growth accelerating, and I see a legacy forming. That's the fuel that keeps me fighting through tough rounds.

If I Do Not Achieve the Goal (£300,000+ in 2025):

- **Lifestyle & Security:** Persistent worries about money, health, and stability. Uncertainty and stress linger as unforeseen expenses threaten my peace of mind.
- **Family & Love:** Travel and celebratory milestones may remain out of reach or scaled back. The lavish experiences and supportive gestures I dreamed of for my loved ones might be postponed or reduced.
- **Professional Investment:** Plans to produce books, enhance Champ Camp, and streamline my business systems could stall due to limited resources, curbing my reach and stalling my professional growth.
- **Legacy & Impact:** With fewer financial resources, my ability to inspire and support charities, the Church, or my community diminishes. The message of what's possible is weakened when resources are scarce.
- **Freedom & Options:** Scarcity restricts my choices—fewer opportunities to improve my personal well-being, assist family members, or indulge in the milestones and rewards I envisioned.

The dreams of elevating my lifestyle and helping others remain constrained by financial limitations.

Activities: Map the Road to Victory

Goals without action are fantasies. In boxing, winning isn't about wanting it more—it's about throwing the right punches at the right time. For a £300,000 turnover, I need daily, weekly, and monthly activities that push me closer to the mark.

Daily Habits:

- **Content Creation:** Delegate 5 pieces of content daily across social platforms, each with a call-to-action (CTA). Content drives awareness, nurtures the audience, and leads to conversions.
- **Lead Generation:** Collect 25 pieces of data (emails, phone numbers) each day. Building a pipeline ensures a steady flow of potential clients.
- **Outreach & Follow-Ups:** Book 5 calls or meetings daily. Whether it's potential clients, sponsors, or partners, consistent outreach drives sales.

Weekly/Monthly Activities:

- **Partnership Outreach:** Aim to secure 3 clients, members, sponsors, or partners per week through scheduled meetings. If I sign 3 a week, that's over 150 deals in a year—even if only a fraction yield substantial revenue, it's progress.
- **Marketing Funnel Optimization:** Every month, review conversion rates, ad performance, and content engagement. Tweak what's not working and double down on what is.
- **Key Results Club Promotion:** Launch monthly promotions to boost Iron, Gold, and Diamond memberships. Offer

discounts, exclusive webinars, or Q&A sessions to entice new sign-ups.
- **Book Sales Strategy:** Each quarter, run a special campaign—like a new book launch, a holiday sale, or a bundle deal—aimed at hitting my volume targets.

Quarterly Check-Ins:

- **Financial Review:** Every quarter, measure progress against the £30k, £100k, £150k checkpoints. If I'm behind, where can I adjust? If I'm ahead, can I invest more into growth?
- **Content & Brand Review:** Evaluate what types of content or promotions are yielding the best returns. Maybe YouTube is crushing it with views but conversions are low—time to add stronger CTAs.

This structured approach ensures I'm not just hoping for revenue; I'm engineering it. I'm training like a fighter—every jab (content), every hook (meetings), and every combination (marketing campaigns) is planned and intentional.

Leverage: Harnessing Resources, People, and Communities

No champion wins alone. Even in boxing, a solitary sport, fighters have trainers, cutmen, sparring partners, and mentors. In business, leverage is about using people, tools, and communities to accelerate growth.

People:

- **Jonathan Reid:** Accountability partner who checks my progress weekly, ensures I don't slack off, and gives honest feedback.

- **Paul O'Mahony:** Skilled in business systems and Facebook ads. His expertise can streamline my marketing funnel and help me convert leads efficiently.
- **Matt Fiddes:** An entrepreneur with a community in health and wealth. His network might open doors to potential clients or partnerships.
- **Freelancer:** Consistent branding and visually appealing marketing materials make a massive difference in credibility and conversions.
- **Romain Neyses:** Maybe a friend outside my business sphere, but supportive in a personal way, reminding me to stay grounded and remember who I am beyond the numbers.

Resources:

- **RSM Online & Acquisition.com (Alex Hormozi):** Educational platforms offering tactics on scaling businesses, improving offers, and maximizing revenues.
- **Instagram Ads, Zoom, Eventbrite, ClickFunnels, Kit.com, iPhone, Youtube, Networking spaces:** Each tool plays a role—Ads to reach new audiences, Zoom for remote consulting calls, Eventbrite for hosting paid workshops, ClickFunnels for sales pages, and my iPhone for on-the-go content creation.

Community:

- **MF Health & Wealth, Health Clubs, Boxing Gyms, Church, Business Networking Groups:** These communities are breeding grounds for trust, referrals, and potential clients. Attending events, masterminds, or simply participating in group discussions can lead to unexpected opportunities.

Leverage ensures I'm not relying solely on my own effort. I'm tapping into collective intelligence, proven strategies, and existing audiences to multiply my effectiveness.

Score: Track, Measure, and Adjust

A boxer watches fight tapes, counts landed punches, and tracks stamina. In business, scoring means tracking KPIs and metrics to know if I'm on course.

Lead KPIs:

- **Content Output:** 5 pieces of content daily.
- **Data Collected:** 25 leads daily.
- **Calls Made**: 25 contacts daily
- **Calls Booked:** 5 calls/meetings daily.

These are activities I can control. If I'm consistent, they'll predict my revenue growth.

Lag KPIs:

- **Monthly Revenue:** Am I hitting £30k in a month at some point? Am I reaching my quarterly targets toward £300k total?
- **Total Clients Signed:** How many Iron, Gold, and Diamond members do I have? How many book sales per month?
- **YouTube Views:** Are we on track for 100 million views across the year?

Review Schedule:

- **Weekly:** Check lead KPIs. Am I posting enough content? Collecting enough leads? Booking enough calls?
- **Monthly:** Assess conversions—are leads turning into clients? Are clients converting into revenue?

- **Quarterly:** Check if I'm reaching major revenue checkpoints. If I'm off track, which part of the funnel needs attention?

Celebration & Adjustments:

- **Hitting the £30k mark:** Treat myself to a nice dinner and a short weekend trip.
- **Reaching £100k:** Invest in a new piece of equipment and take my family out to celebrate.
- **At £300k:** This calls for a significant celebration—maybe that watch I've wanted, a donation to my church or a mental health charity, and a family gathering to savor the moment.

Scoring keeps me honest. Without data, I'm guessing. With data, I'm strategising. Great fighters adapt round by round, and I will adapt month by month to ensure I'm inching closer to that £300k finish line.

Personal Stories and Champion Quotes

I remember early in my career, when generating a few thousand pounds felt like a big deal. I had no systems, just raw hustle. Over time, I learned from mentors who'd done six figures, then seven, and they all said the same thing: success leaves clues. Tony Robbins hammered into me the importance of modeling success. Jordan Belfort showed me how to refine my sales pitch and close deals ethically and effectively. Paul O'Mahony reinforced the power of digital marketing funnels.

These lessons are like the coaches in a fighter's corner. Mike Tyson had Cus D'Amato whispering wisdom and strategy. Muhammed Ali believed in himself to the point of prophecy, declaring he was "The Greatest" long before the world agreed. Their conviction and guidance shaped their paths. I draw from that energy—believing fully in the £300k goal, knowing I can get there with the right moves.

In love and family, there's inspiration too. Consider entrepreneurs who balance massive income goals with a rich family life. They show that wealth can coexist with happiness, humility, and helping others. If David Goggins can push his body beyond conceivable limits and James Clear can break down massive goals into tiny habits, I can break £300k into daily tasks and monthly milestones.

Applying the 12 Key Principles of Success

Throughout this book, I've emphasised principles: faith, vision, teamwork, focus, hard work & dedication, discipline, the will to win, resilience, confidence, respect, humility, and legacy. Generating £300,000 aligns perfectly:

- **Faith:** I believe I can achieve this even before the proof emerges.
- **Vision:** The outcome is crystal clear—£300k by year-end.
- **Teamwork:** I'm leveraging people, resources, and communities.
- **Focus:** Daily content, daily leads, daily calls—no slacking.
- **Hard Work & Dedication:** Posting content at midnight if needed, making calls even on tough days.
- **Discipline:** Sticking to the plan even when I don't feel like it.
- **The Will to Win:** Embracing setbacks as stepping stones, not stumbling blocks.
- **Resilience:** If a campaign fails, I'll refine it and come back stronger.
- **Confidence:** I've done it before in other contexts, I can do it again now.
- **Respect:** Treat clients, partners, and audiences with integrity, ensuring long-term relationships.
- **Humility:** Acknowledging I don't have all answers, seeking mentorship, and constantly learning.
- **Legacy:** Beyond the numbers, £300k means leaving a footprint—changing lives, inspiring others, and building a future legacy for my family.

Taking the First Steps

The moment I publish this chapter, the clock starts ticking. January 1, 2025, begins the journey, and December 31 closes it. In that time, I'll have faced challenges—maybe some months won't hit targets, maybe a deal falls through. That's part of the fight.

But I know this: every day I train, every piece of content I post, every call I make, and every meeting I secure moves me closer. Consistency breaks mountains. In boxing, relentless training turns a novice into a contender. In business, relentless activity and refinement turn a small-time coach into a major player.

I recall a time when I struggled to make even £1,000 in a month. I thought I lacked something fundamental—maybe I wasn't cut out for entrepreneurship. Then I learned to treat it like boxing: train, learn, measure, adapt, and never give up. Six months later, I hit £10,000 in a month. That taught me a crucial lesson: growth is exponential once you find your groove. If I can go from £1,000 to £10,000, I can go from £10,000 to £300,000 with the right plan, mindset, and execution.

Your Turn: Invest 12 Minutes

Now it's your turn. You might not have a £300,000 target. Maybe it's £30,000 or £3 million. Maybe it's not money at all—maybe it's a different kind of goal. The principles remain the same.

Take 12 minutes now to:

1. **Write Your Gratitude List:** Identify at least 5 things that support your goal.
2. **Define Your Outcome:** Make it SMART, break it into checkpoints, and clarify why it matters.
3. **List Your Activities:** Daily, weekly, monthly—what steps will drive you forward?
4. **Identify Leverage:** Who can help you? What tools or communities can boost your progress?

5. **Set Up Your Scoring System:** Choose KPIs, schedule reviews, and plan celebrations.

Don't overthink—just start. Write it down, refine later. This simple exercise transforms your dream from a distant wish into a plan of action.

Stepping Into the Ring of Opportunity

Generating £300,000 in annual turnover isn't just about money. It's a symbol of personal growth, the impact I can create, and the legacy I'm building. It's a mile marker on my journey from unplanned paths to clear designs.

In boxing, stepping into the ring takes courage, training, and a belief in your ability to triumph. In business and life, the same holds true. With clarity, action, support, and tracking, I can—and will—achieve this goal.

Remember, as the Boxing Life Coach, I'm not just telling you what to do; I'm doing it myself. We're in this fight together—using the same principles, sharing the same struggles, and celebrating the same victories.

Now, lace up your gloves. Your championship fight—a better life, bigger goals, bold dreams—awaits.

10

Publish 33 Books

When I think about publishing 33 books in a single year, I'm reminded of the sheer determination required to step into the ring as an underdog. Most people never even dream of writing one book, let alone dozens. I've learned that turning dreams into reality isn't just about grand statements—it's about daily actions, unwavering focus, and a hunger to achieve what most consider impossible.

Like mastering a new boxing combination, writing and publishing so many books demands discipline, creativity, and a willingness to push beyond comfort zones. Each book isn't just another title; it's a building block for my legacy, a stepping stone towards authority, impact, and financial freedom. Just as a champion fighter embraces the toughest training to outlast competitors, I must embrace a rigorous writing routine to outpace average results. A space of creativity where I leverage ideas, AI, and the network of amazing people I can learn from to deliver pieces of art. Each book will grip readers in a different way. A year by design and 12 boxing principles of success are building blocks which the other 31 books will come off from. A set of book series that will inspire, motivate and empower dreamers and high achievers to fight for success for centuries to come. This is more than a mission, it is a movement.

By applying the GOALS framework—Gratitude, Outcome, Activities, Leverage, and Score—I can transform this daunting ambition into an actionable blueprint.

Gratitude: The Foundation of Strength

Before I embark on this year-long literary journey, I remind myself of what I'm grateful for, grounding me in positivity:

1. **Past Experience:** I've published 2 books before. I know the feeling of taking an idea to a finished product, and that experience shortens the learning curve this time around.
2. **Love of Reading:** My passion for reading fuels my creativity. Just as a fighter studies legends to refine technique, I've studied countless authors to learn storytelling and structure.
3. **Prolific Reading History:** I've read over 33 books in the past year, absorbing diverse writing styles and narrative techniques that I can now apply in my own work.
4. **No Direct Comparison:** I haven't met someone who has published 33 books in a year. This means I'm charting new territory, defining what's possible rather than following someone else's path.
5. **Historical Precedent:** While the exact timeframe differs, authors like Emily Brontë and L. Ron Hubbard produced enormous bodies of work. Their prolific output proves that high-volume publishing can be done.

Gratitude keeps me focused and humble. Just as a boxer appreciates every round of sparring, I appreciate every lesson, mentor, and experience that brought me here. My gratitude reminds me that I'm not starting from scratch—I'm starting from a position of strength.

Outcome: Defining the Target & Understanding the Stakes
SMART Goal:
I will publish 33 books by May 27, 2025.

- **Specific:** Exactly 33 titles, each fully published and released.

- **Measurable:** Count the books—either I hit 33 or I don't.
- **Achievable:** Ambitious yet feasible with the right systems, discipline, and consistent writing.
- **Relevant:** Aligns perfectly with my role as a Super Author, boosting my brand and audience reach.
- **Time-Bound:** With a deadline of May 27, 2025, I have a clear finish line that creates urgency.

List of the 33 Books:

1. 12 Boxing Principles of Success (2nd edition - done)
2. A Year by Design
3. Turning Goals to Reality (Series x 5)
4. Train Like a Fighter (Series x 5)
5. Think Like a Champion (Series x 5)
6. Level Up Like a Boss (Series x 5)
7. Champions of Christ (Series x 5)
8. Super Author
9. Key Results Club
10. Stories of Success: Key Black Figures
11. 20/25
12. Make Memories in Marbella
13. Make Memories in London
14. First Team Dream
15. Fit Over Fifty
16. The Datemeister
17. Marriage Manifestation
18. Boxing Combinations
19. Champion Transformations
20. 10K Level Up Challenge
21. 100 Affirmations
22. 100 Goals
23. 100 Visualisation Techniques

24. The Jab
25. Elite Super Strength Endurance
26. A Book of Quotes for Success
27. Quotes from the Greats
28. A to Z of Boxing
29. Turning Goals to Reality
30. Boss Up & Ball - Unique Partnerships

There are more than 33 books that make this list so I will select from this list. I am not limited to these book titles as since I've been working on this book, more ideas have come into fruition that are more time sensitive. The list above contains the majority of my titles but not all.

Checkpoints:

- **10 Books Published:** Confirms early momentum and feasibility.
- **22 Books Published:** Over two-thirds complete, proving sustained productivity.
- **33 Books Published:** The final victory, showing I achieved the ambitious target.

My Why
If I Achieve the Goal (33 Books Published):

- **Authority & Legacy:** I become a leading figure in my field, leaving behind a body of work that outlasts me and inspires countless readers.
- **Financial Gain & Brand Recognition:** More titles mean multiple income streams, a stronger personal brand, and increased revenue through book sales, royalties, and related products.

- **Audience Growth & Credibility:** Each book attracts new readers, broadening my influence and making me a go-to expert. My words can shape opinions, guide personal transformations, and ignite dreams.
- **Professional Opportunities:** Increased networking possibilities, speaking engagements, and collaborations with top-tier industry players become accessible. Media outlets and event organizers take note, respecting my prolific output.
- **Personal Fulfillment & Confidence:** Overcoming this monumental challenge strengthens my self-belief. Achieving something so rare proves that no goal is too big if approached with discipline and vision.
- **Creativity, Knowledge & Mastery:** Writing 33 books sharpens my storytelling, research, and narrative skills. I become more resourceful, insightful, and effective, not just as a writer but as a business leader and coach.
- **Global Reach & Cultural Impact:** Digital platforms enable worldwide distribution, spreading my ideas, lessons, and stories to audiences I've never met, leaving a footprint in global conversations.
- **Lasting Example for Loved Ones:** Creating this library of work sets a standard of excellence for my family and future generations, showing them what relentless pursuit of a goal can accomplish.

If I Do Not Achieve the Goal (Failing to Reach 33 Books):

- **Unrealised Potential:** I miss out on proving what's possible, settling for mediocrity instead of extraordinary achievement.
- **Reduced Impact & Influence:** With fewer titles, my authority, audience reach, and credibility remain limited. Readers have less reason to see me as a thought leader, and my messages resonate with fewer people.

- **Fewer Professional Opportunities:** I might struggle to stand out in a crowded marketplace, limiting media exposure, speaking gigs, and collaborations that could have accelerated my career.
- **Lower Confidence & Momentum:** Missing the target can dampen my self-belief, making future ambitious goals seem harder to achieve.
- **Lost Legacy & Cultural Contribution:** Without a rich catalog, I leave behind less for future readers, diminishing my ability to shape narratives, opinions, and lives.
- **Creative Stagnation:** Producing fewer books means less practice, potentially stunting my growth as a writer. My understanding of storytelling and idea execution may not reach its full potential.

Just like a championship fight, the stakes are high. Victory brings power, influence, and inspiration. Defeat means unrealised dreams and fewer opportunities to lead, teach, and inspire. Understanding both scenarios fuels my commitment to see this through.

Activities: The Daily, Weekly, and Monthly Grind

Ambitious goals are achieved through daily actions. As a boxer trains daily to hone skills, I must write regularly and manage production efficiently.

Publishing Process Steps:

1. **Plan the Book:** Decide title, outline table of contents, and envision the cover.
2. **Prepare Content:** Research, interview if needed, and gather material.
3. **Write Manuscript:** Draft chapters, aiming for clarity and engagement.

4. **Edit & Format:** Refine the manuscript, format for print and digital versions, and secure cover art.
5. **Launch & Market:** Promote the book, seek reviews, run deals, and integrate it into my brand strategy.

1. **Plan the Book:** Decide title, outline, table of contents, and cover draft.
2. **Prepare Content:** Research (interview if needed), Write, and Edit.
3. **Publish Manuscript:** Format, Illustrate, Upload & Order

Launch & Market: Once I have completed the 3 steps above, I can begin promoting the book, seeking reviews, securing unique partnerships, and integrate them into my brand strategy.

Daily Habits:

- Write for 1 hour each day, focusing on drafting or refining chapters.
- On weekends, add an extra 4-hour writing block. This totals about 6 hours per week dedicated to book creation and production.

Monthly Targets & Adaptations:

- Aim to draft at least 7 books per month.
- If I'm falling behind, consider increasing daily writing time to 2 hours or outsourcing certain tasks like editing or cover design.
- Utilise dictation software and AI prompts for first drafts to speed up writing.

By breaking the massive goal into actionable steps, I ensure steady progress. Each chapter written is a jab landed, each finished manuscript another round won, and each published book a victory declared.

Leverage: Utilising Resources, People, and Communities

Champions don't go it alone. They have trainers, managers, and mentors. I'll tap into people, tools, and networks that accelerate my publishing journey.

People:

- **Jonathan Reid (Accountability Partner):** Weekly check-ins to track how many chapters or drafts I've completed.
- **Gerry Robert & Tunji Olunjimi (Book Systems Experts):** Their proven methods can streamline my production, marketing, and distribution.
- **Freelancers:** Professional covers, editors and graphic designers for formatting and publishing to ensure each book looks polished and professional.

Resources:

- **Gerry Robert's site & Daniel Priestley's Guides:** For marketing tactics, bulk sales, and international reach.
- **"Publish a Book and Grow Rich" & IngramSpark, Nielsen:** Distribution platforms and technical guidance for ISBN, print, and eBook formats.

Communities:

- **MF Health & Wealth, Black Business Book Festival, David Lloyd Club:** Networking with other authors, sharing insights, gaining support and moral encouragement.

Leverage means I'm not fighting this match alone. I have corner men, strategic partners, and mentors guiding me. Just as a fighter learns from a skilled coach, I'll learn from experts who've navigated publishing before.

Score: Tracking Progress & Celebrating Milestones

In boxing, you count rounds, punches, and victories. For writing, I must measure writing time, drafts completed, and books published.

Lead KPIs (Process Indicators):

- **Daily Writing Time:** Did I write for at least 1 hour today?
- **Drafts Completed:** How many manuscripts are in draft form this month?
- **Editing Sessions:** How many chapters have I polished this week?

Lag KPIs (Result Indicators):

- **Books Published:** Am I hitting the checkpoints—10, then 22, then 33?
- **Monthly Release Count:** How many books go live each month or quarter?

Review Schedule:

- **Weekly:** Check if I wrote daily and advanced any manuscripts closer to completion.
- **Monthly:** Ensure I'm meeting monthly publishing targets (around 7 books per month).
- **Quarterly:** Assess progress against the first 10, then 22 published milestones.

Celebrate Wins:

- At 10 Books: Treat myself to a nice dinner or a small getaway.
- At 22 Books: Maybe invest in something that boosts productivity or well-being, such as ergonomic furniture or a relaxation retreat.
- At 33 Books: A grand celebration—an event with family and friends, possibly a high-end watch or another symbolic reward that reminds me of this victory.

Adjust if necessary. If I'm behind schedule after the first quarter, I might add extra writing hours or outsource formatting. Like a boxer switching strategy mid-match, I remain agile and responsive to feedback.

Personal Stories & Inspirational Quotes

I remember the struggle of finishing my very first book. It felt like climbing a mountain. Now, aiming for 33, I'm scaling Everest. Yet, every legendary champion—from Muhammad Ali to Mike Tyson—faced insurmountable odds and overcame them by turning massive dreams into step-by-step plans.

In love, life, and business, I've seen people who took on epic challenges and succeeded because they refused to accept limitations. Consider entrepreneurs who launched multiple products in a year, or athletes who completed multiple marathons. Their stories prove that extraordinary feats are possible.

As a Boxing Life Coach, I'm blending that fighter's mindset with the author's pen. I'm rewriting the narrative of what it means to be prolific. When Emily Brontë or L. Ron Hubbard wrote prolifically, they left cultural imprints. I aim to do the same—my pages filled with wisdom, inspiration, and stories that guide others on their own journeys.

Applying the 12 Key Principles of Success

This entire endeavor exemplifies the 12 key principles: faith, vision, teamwork, focus, hard work & dedication, discipline, the will to win, resilience, confidence, respect, humility, and legacy.

- **Faith:** Believing I can accomplish what few even attempt.
- **Vision:** Seeing 33 completed books, each serving a purpose.
- **Teamwork:** Leveraging coaches, designers, editors, and communities.
- **Focus:** Sticking to daily writing goals despite distractions.
- **Hard Work & Dedication:** Showing up day after day, word after word.
- **Discipline:** Maintaining a writing schedule, even on tough days.
- **The Will to Win:** Embracing challenges and pushing through obstacles.
- **Resilience:** Bouncing back when a manuscript proves difficult or a day is missed.
- **Confidence:** Trusting my abilities, honed by past success and experience.
- **Respect:** Respecting the craft, my readers, and the process.
- **Humility:** Knowing there's always more to learn and improve.
- **Legacy:** Leaving a body of work that inspires, educates, and empowers others long after I'm gone.

Your Turn: Invest 12 Minutes

Take 12 minutes now to:

1. **Define Your Own Writing Goal:** Maybe it's one book this year or a blog series, or a podcast —make it SMART.

2. **Write Your Why:** What happens if you achieve it? What if you don't?
3. **List Daily Activities:** How much time will you dedicate to writing each day or week?
4. **Find Leverage:** Who can help you? What resources or communities will accelerate your progress?
5. **Set KPIs:** How will you measure success along the way?

Don't overthink—just start writing. Progress begins the moment you commit.

Becoming a Prolific Champion

Publishing 33 books in a year is no different than aiming for a world title in boxing. It's about daring greatly, committing fully, and executing consistently. I have gratitude in my corner, a clear outcome in my sights, activities defined, leverage lined up, and a scoring system to keep me honest.

This journey isn't just about the number 33—it's about becoming the kind of person who can achieve something so extraordinary. It's about proving to myself and others that with the right mindset, strategy, and discipline, impossible dreams can become inevitable realities.

As I put pen to paper, I'm not just writing pages—I'm writing a legacy of resilience, ambition, and unwavering belief. Each book I publish is another round won, another opponent bested, and another testament to the power of turning dreams into action.

As the Boxing Life Coach, I want you to know that you, too, can tackle outlandish goals. You can become the champion of your own story. The 12 key principles are your cornermen, the GOALS framework, your fight strategy. Your first draft is the opening bell.

The arena is set. The crowd waits. Let's put pen to paper, one book at a time, until 33 stand tall on the shelves—living proof of what happens when you design your year and live it with purpose, grit, and unstoppable determination.

11

Make Memories With My Girlfriend

When it comes to building a loving, lasting relationship—one that leads to marriage, children, and a lifetime of shared joy—you can't just rely on chance. Like training for a championship fight, meaningful connection requires intention, strategy, and consistent effort. I want to make memories weekly with my girlfriend, but first I must find her, show genuine interest, nurture a deep bond, and ensure we always have something special to look forward to each week.

This chapter is about designing a plan for love just as I'd design a plan for business growth or athletic success. Instead of leaving it to luck, I'm going to apply the GOALS framework—Gratitude, Outcome, Activities, Leverage, and Score—to transform the abstract idea of "making weekly memories" into a concrete, achievable reality. Just as a boxer commits to daily training, I'll commit to weekly adventures and intentional steps towards finding and cherishing memories with the right partner.

Gratitude: Starting from a Place of Strength

Before I set out to create these memories, I acknowledge what I have going for me:

1. **Past Experience:** I've had girlfriends before, learning valuable lessons about what I want in a relationship and how to communicate better.
2. **Abundant Opportunities:** There are Millions of women 25+ who are also seeking meaningful connections. There's no scarcity of potential partners.
3. **My Health & Fitness:** I'm strong, fit, and healthy, which contributes to my confidence and energy—qualities that help me fully engage in memorable activities.
4. **Personality & Charisma:** I'm funny, charismatic, and can connect on multiple levels—mentally, spiritually, physically, sexually—which helps me stand out.
5. **Growth Mindset:** I've learned from personal development and boxing: I can improve my relationship skills, attract the right woman, and build a stable, loving home life.

Gratitude grounds me. Just as a fighter appreciates every sparring partner, I appreciate every experience and attribute that positions me to find love and cultivate it through weekly shared memories.

Outcome: Defining the Goal & Understanding Its Stakes
SMART Goal:

I will make memories weekly with my girlfriend. This involves three phases:

1. Creating memorable moments each week as a single man, making memories, meeting new people and exploring activities.
2. Dating and connecting with women, building rapport and compatibility until I find a partner who aligns with my vision.
3. Once committed, continuing to make weekly memories as a couple, strengthening our bond and preparing for a future with marriage and children.

Checkpoints:

1. Make memories weekly as a single man.
2. Date beautiful, compatible women regularly.
3. Commit to the woman I see a future with—someone who wants marriage and kids.
4. Continue making weekly memories as a committed couple, laying the foundation for family life.

My Why
If I Achieve the Goal (Making Weekly Memories With My Girlfriend):

1. **Emotional Bond & Best-Friend Connection:**
   By sharing adventures each week, we deepen our understanding and trust, transforming our relationship into a genuine partnership where she becomes my closest confidante.
2. **Family Foundation & Future Stability:**
   Consistent quality time and growing intimacy set the stage for marriage and children. We're not just dating; we're building a home where our future kids will witness love, teamwork, and respect.
3. **Relationship Growth & Long-Term Happiness:**
   Regular positive experiences prevent stagnation, keeping romance alive and ensuring we evolve as a couple. This leads to a more stable, fulfilling relationship that stands the test of time.
4. **Shared Purpose & Vision:**
   Weekly memories help us align on long-term goals—whether it's buying a home, traveling the world, or raising children who learn from our example. We create a shared narrative of what life can be.

5. **Cultural & Intellectual Enrichment:**
   By trying new activities—museums, concerts, workshops—we both become more well-rounded individuals. This enrichment benefits our future family, as we'll pass on curiosity, creativity, and open-mindedness to our children.

If I Do Not Achieve the Goal (Not Making Weekly Memories):

1. **Emotional Distance & Stagnation:**
   Without regular bonding, we risk drifting apart, losing that special spark and intimate understanding. The relationship may feel dull, and love may fade into routine.
2. **Weaker Foundation for the Future:**
   Without shared experiences, committing to marriage and planning for children becomes uncertain. The lack of a strong emotional base makes discussions about long-term life goals feel forced.
3. **Lower Relationship Satisfaction & Greater Vulnerability:**
   Without consistent positive interactions, dissatisfaction can brew. This might increase misunderstandings or even the likelihood of breakups, as neither partner feels truly valued or understood.
4. **Fewer Shared Adventures & Limited Growth:**
   Without exploring new activities, we miss opportunities to learn together, grow as individuals, and inspire each other. Life becomes static, offering little to look forward to each week.
5. **Reduced Inspiration & Legacy:**
   Without cherished memories, we have fewer stories to pass on to our children. We miss the chance to model love, cooperation, and a zest for life—lessening the impact and legacy we could leave behind.

Understanding these two scenarios keeps me motivated. Just as a boxer imagines both victory and defeat before a match, I envision the warmth of a loving home filled with laughter versus the emptiness of a love that never fully blossomed. The stakes are high, and I'm determined to make each week count.

Activities: Daily, Weekly, and Monthly Habits

To achieve this, I need a plan that ensures consistent action and progress. Like training drills for a boxer, I'll establish habits that make finding and nurturing a relationship inevitable.

Phases:

1. **Single & Mingling:**
   Spend time on my own making great memories doing what I love, meeting people on the way. These activities include: Working Out, Relaxing, Reading, Learning, Playing, Laughing, Dancing, Singing, Listening, Traveling, Watching, Digesting(Food & Drink). **Dating & Selection:**
   Approach attractive women, offer genuine compliments, ask interesting questions, and introduce yourself. Invite them to join you on a memory making moment, mission or movement. A moment is a brief 300 second catch up consisting of single & mingling activities. A mission is 300 minutes of single & mingling activities. A movement is 300 hours of single & mingling activities.

2. **Committed Relationship:**
   Once I find a woman who I love spending time with and shares my dreams of marriage and family, we will continue the weekly memory-making ritual—exploring restaurants, traveling, attending concerts, watching sunsets, listening to the birds sing, learning new skills together.

For example:

- **Fridays:** A 3-hour evening window for a low-pressure outing—could be a local jazz bar or a museum event.
- **Saturdays (4 pm - 10 pm):** Date night slot—dinner, a movie, salsa lessons, or a comedy club.
- **Sundays (3 pm - 8 pm):** Daytime adventures—brunch, a hiking trip, visiting a farmers' market, or attending a cultural festival.

By pre-scheduling these times, I ensure consistency. Like a fighter dedicating certain days to cardio or sparring, I dedicate certain periods to social and romantic growth.

Leverage: Utilising People, Resources, and Communities

No champion rises alone. I need mentors, guides, and communities to support my journey from single life to a committed relationship.

People:

- **Justina Omotayo (Accountability Partner):** We can check in weekly to ensure I'm sticking to the plan if single, or maintained weekly memories if coupled.
- **Dating Coches & Gurus:** For guidance on emotional intimacy and communication, helping me connect on deeper levels.
- **Neil Strauss (Author of "The Game"):** His insights can encourage me to step outside my comfort zone, refine my social skills, and approach dating more confidently.

Resources:

- **The Game, Rules of the Game:** Practical guidelines for social dynamics and connecting with women authentically.

- **Hinge & Eventbrite:** Hinge for online dating leads; Eventbrite for discovering workshops, cultural events, and mixers to meet new people.
- **Love Languages Knowledge:** Understanding the 5 love languages helps me communicate affection in a way that resonates with each woman I meet.

Communities:

- **Health Clubs & Gyms:** Meeting fitness-oriented individuals who value health and energy.
- **Church & Workshops:** Connecting with people who share spiritual or cultural values, potentially meeting someone with similar life goals.
- **Instagram & Library Events:** Social media challenges or book clubs to spark conversations and find like-minded people.

Like a fighter with coaches and a support team, I'm leveraging networks and resources to make the dating process smoother and more rewarding.

Score: Tracking Progress & Celebrating Wins

In the boxing ring, you count landed punches, track endurance, and review footage. In building a love life, I must track metrics that show progress.

Lead KPIs (Actions I Control):

- **5 Activities Completed Weekly:** Ensure I'm consistently engaging in social or cultural experiences.
- **25 Compliments to Women Weekly:** Compliments are icebreakers, encouraging me to approach and engage.
- **5 Women Asked Out Weekly (If Single):** Keeps me proactive in meeting potential partners.

- **2 Dates Weekly (Once Dating):** Ensures I'm giving myself enough opportunities to find the right match.

Lag KPIs (Results I Aim For):

- **Committed Relationship:** Eventually, I aim to find a girlfriend who shares my vision of marriage and family.
- **Consistent Weekly Memories as a Couple:** Once committed, track that we never skip a week without a meaningful activity.

Review Schedule:

- **Weekly:** Check if I met my activity and compliment quotas.
- **Monthly:** Evaluate quality of connections—am I meeting women who inspire me and share my future plans?
- **Quarterly:** Assess if I'm closer to finding the right partner. If not, do I need to change my approach, attend different events, or refine my conversation skills?

Celebration & Adjustments:

- **Initial Wins:** When I start having regular dates or begin to see one woman consistently, treat myself to something small—a nice meal or a new book.
- **Relationship Start:** When I commit to a girlfriend who shares my vision, celebrate with a special weekend trip or a unique experience that marks the new chapter.
- **Continual Memories:** Each quarter, review highlights, maybe creating a photo album or journal, reinforcing how far I've come.

If I'm not hitting targets, I'll adjust strategies—try new communities, hire a dating coach, or spend more time learning about body language and building long term relationships. Like a boxer refining technique mid-tournament, I stay flexible and determined.

Personal Stories & Inspirational Quotes

I remember a time when I felt too shy to approach someone I found attractive. Over time, I practiced just like a boxer drills footwork. I learned to be genuine, to compliment sincerely, and to ask confidently. Each small success built my courage.

Muhammad Ali believed in himself long before the world recognized him as "The Greatest." That faith in one's abilities applies to romance, too. I must believe that I can find the right partner and build a life that includes love, family, and weekly adventures.

I've seen entrepreneurs approach their love lives with the same strategic thinking they apply to their businesses—setting goals, learning communication techniques, making time for connection. Their relationships thrived because they treated love like a priority, not an afterthought.

As the Boxing Life Coach, I know that discipline, commitment, and authenticity are as essential in love as they are in boxing or business. The 12 key principles I rely on for personal development and boxing training also guide my romantic journey.

Applying the 12 Key Principles of Success

- **Faith:** Believing I can attract a woman who shares my values and dreams.
- **Vision:** Envisioning a future where we marry, have children, and grow old together with stories to tell.
- **Teamwork:** Working together to create a unified front, supporting each other's growth and dreams.
- **Focus:** Regularly planning activities, never letting weeks pass by without investing in connection.

- **Hard Work & Dedication:** Overcoming social fears, staying consistent in compliments, invites, and follow-ups.
- **Discipline:** Sticking to my schedule of weekly activities and dates, even when life gets busy.
- **The Will to Win:** Persisting despite rejections or unsuccessful dates, knowing the right partner awaits.
- **Resilience:** Bouncing back if a promising connection doesn't pan out, learning from each experience.
- **Confidence:** Trusting my worth, character, and capacity to offer love and stability.
- **Respect:** Treating every woman with kindness, understanding boundaries, and listening carefully.
- **Humility:** Recognising I have more to learn about relationships, staying open to advice and growth.
- **Legacy:** Imagining the family we'll build, the lessons we'll pass on, and the loving example we'll set for our children.

Your Turn: Invest 12 Minutes
Take 12 minutes now:

1. **Define Your Relationship Goal:** Maybe it's one meaningful date a week or reconnecting deeply with your current partner.
2. **Write Your Why:** What happens if you achieve or don't achieve this relationship vision?
3. **List Activities:** Brainstorm fun, varied experiences to share—movies, hikes, museums, dance lessons.
4. **Identify Leverage:** Who can guide you—friends, a coach, a book? Which communities or apps can help you meet new people?
5. **Set KPIs:** How many activities, compliments, invites, or dates per week?

Don't overthink—just start. Like throwing your first jab in the gym, that initial step leads to growth.

Designing a Love Story One Week at a Time

Making weekly memories with my girlfriend is about more than romance—it's about building a life together, preparing for marriage, and laying the groundwork for children who grow up in a loving, stable home.

Like a fighter who trains daily, I will approach love with discipline, strategy, and heart. By applying gratitude, setting clear outcomes, committing to regular activities, leveraging support, and tracking my progress, I transform the dream of finding and nurturing my life partner into a guided journey.

This is my fight for love, family, and legacy. With dedication, I will create stories worth telling, and one day, my children will smile as I share the tale of how I met their mother, and we built our love, one weekly memory at a time.

12

Celebrate Success with Family & Friends

If I've learned anything through my years of training, it's that no fighter truly wins alone. Behind every champion, there's a team—family, friends, mentors, and supporters—who stand in the corner, patching wounds, cheering wildly, and celebrating each victory as if it were their own. You might step into the ring by yourself, but you never step out alone. And that spirit of communal triumph isn't limited to boxing. Whether we're talking about birthdays, weddings, or personal milestones like promotions or moving abroad, true success is best savored when it's shared.

In this chapter, we'll explore why celebrating success with family and friends is not just a "nice thing to do," but a critical component of a life well-lived. Think of it as the final round of your achievement—raising your arms high, looking around, and seeing the faces of those who believed in you all along.

What Qualifies as "Success"?

Success isn't a one-size-fits-all concept. A newlywed is celebrating the merging of two families; a fresh graduate is celebrating the conclusion of a demanding academic journey; a business owner might be celebrating the first profitable quarter. I like to keep it simple by focusing on the big three:

1. **Birthdays:** Each birthday is a milestone marking another year of growth, lessons learned, and experiences gained.
2. **Weddings:** A day of ultimate commitment, merging dreams and futures—a powerhouse moment that deserves communal joy.
3. **Big Wins (Promotions, Moving Abroad, Completing a Challenge):** These can take many forms—a new job title, the excitement of starting life in a foreign country, or finally crossing the finish line in a personal challenge.

I've chosen to emphasise these events, but the principle of celebration applies universally. It could be completing a fitness program, organising a community fundraiser, or conquering a fear you've had for years. Success is success—even if it's a success only you and your loved ones fully appreciate.

Being a Good Leader in the Community is also worth celebrating. If you're on a mission to inspire, motivate, and empower others—whether in fitness, business, or day-to-day life—then each step you take toward unity and collective achievement is a win. And wins, my friend, demand applause.

G.O.A.L.S. Framework for Celebration

We'll use the same G.O.A.L.S. framework that's guided other parts of *A Year By Design*:

1. **Gratitude**
2. **Outcome**
3. **Activities**
4. **Leverage**
5. **Score**

Each step ensures we approach celebration with the same intentionality we bring to big business goals or personal feats. After all, celebrating success is just as essential as achieving it.

Gratitude: Honouring the People and Moments That Shape Us

Gratitude is the heartbeat of any celebration. When you reflect on how you reached a milestone—be it a birthday, a wedding, or a major personal win—you'll find an intricate web of people and opportunities that guided your path. Much like a boxer who thanks everyone from the trainer to the person who handles media interviews, we have many behind-the-scenes supporters.

Five Things I'm Grateful For (Towards Celebrating Success):

1. **Loving Family:** My family forms the backbone of my life. Their unconditional support and occasional tough love push me to strive for greatness.
2. **Amazing Friends:** Friends are the siblings we choose. They celebrate our wins, console our losses, and add color to every event we hold.
3. **Surrounded by Driven People:** By associating with motivated, goal-oriented individuals, I'm constantly reminded to keep pushing my limits.
4. **Memorable Celebrations:** Some of my favorite life moments are recorded in photos and videos from birthdays, weddings, or random gatherings. Those memories fuel my spirit.
5. **Opportunities to Celebrate (Birthdays, Weddings, Achievements):** Life's tapestry is woven with these special milestones, each a chance to unite loved ones and share in a deeper bond.

Just as a champion boxer thanks the crowd for their energy, we, too, can express appreciation to the "crowd" of family and friends who stand by our side. Gratitude frames the celebration, reminding us it's about more than a party—it's about honoring the bonds and blessings that carry us.

Outcome: Clarifying the Purpose and Scale of Your Celebration

What exactly are we aiming for when we say "celebrate success with family and friends"? Without clarity, a well-meaning plan can devolve into a half-hearted gathering, or worse, slip off your radar entirely because "other things came up." By defining a SMART objective, you ensure that your celebration is purposeful and impactful.

SMART Celebration Goal

- **Specific:** "I will celebrate success with my family and friends at least once every month, using birthdays, weddings, or major achievements (promotion, moving abroad, completing a challenge) as focal points."
- **Measurable:** "Each month, I'll host or attend an event, big or small, that commemorates at least one milestone within my circle."
- **Achievable:** "I'll focus on realistic events—birthdays, existing traditions, or personal wins. I'll set a manageable budget and time frame."
- **Relevant:** "Celebrating success aligns with my mission to be a good leader in my community, fostering gratitude, humility, and connection among those I love."
- **Time-Bound:** "I'll maintain this monthly celebration schedule throughout 2025, ensuring at least 12 events total."

Why It Matters: My Top Ten Motives for Celebrating

1. **Strengthening Bonds:** Shared joy cements relationships, turning casual acquaintances into lifelong friends.

2. **Maintaining Connections:** In our busy world, it's easy to drift apart. Regular celebrations keep relationships alive.
3. **Balancing Intensity:** This year, I'm working, training, and grinding hard. Celebrations help me exhale and replenish my energy.
4. **Leadership by Example:** If I, a Boxing Life Coach, emphasise communal joy, others realise it's okay—and necessary—to pause and appreciate life.
5. **Family Importance:** Family is a cornerstone. If they see me cherishing milestones, it strengthens our generational legacy.
6. **Friends as Chosen Family:** Friends are the tribe that stands in your corner, championing your dreams.
7. **Inspire Gratitude:** Celebrating fosters an environment of thankfulness and positivity—an antidote to stress.
8. **Spread Positivity:** When we celebrate, we invite others to reflect on their own accomplishments, creating a domino effect of happiness.
9. **Memories to Treasure:** Years down the line, these celebrations will form the highlight reel of my life.
10. **Continual Encouragement:** Each win celebrated acts as a stepping stone for the next goal, fueling ongoing motivation.

Defining your desired outcome clarifies why you're partying in the first place. It's not just to kill time but to bond, rejuvenate, and set an example of balanced living.

What Happens If I Don't Celebrate Success?

Skipping celebration might not seem catastrophic—until you realize what you lose. Below is a five-point breakdown reminiscent of the structure used in previous chapters:

1. **Missed Emotional Bonding:**
Without celebrations, you forfeit opportunities to deepen your

relationships. Over time, this can erode closeness and mutual trust.

2. **Weaker Motivation & Team Spirit:**
Celebrations refuel your emotional tank and everyone else's. Without them, you risk a culture where achievements go unnoticed, breeding apathy.

3. **Unrecognised Support Systems:**
If you don't honour achievements, you also overlook the people who helped you along the way. They may feel their efforts are taken for granted, potentially undermining future collaboration.

4. **Increased Isolation & Burnout:**
Neglecting celebrations can lead you to focus solely on the grind—business, training, or personal challenges—without the relational balm that fosters resilience.

5. **Lost Momentum for Future Goals:**
Celebrations create an uplifting cycle, encouraging bigger ambitions. Without that "victory high," setting and achieving new goals can feel more like drudgery than an exciting journey.

Like a fighter who walks away from the ring without acknowledging the crowd or the corner, you'd be missing a golden chance to stoke community energy and reaffirm your sense of purpose.

Activities: Making Celebration a Habit

Just as I schedule training sessions or business meetings, I must also schedule celebrations. Often, the idea of a party or dinner is overshadowed by day-to-day responsibilities—unless it's integrated into the routine.

Daily, Weekly, Monthly Habits

- **Daily Habit (Micro-Celebrations):** A simple "congratulations" message to someone who achieved something. This could

be as small as finishing a tough workout or acing a job interview. Small, genuine acknowledgments keep positivity alive.
- **Weekly Habit:** Check in on relatives or friends with birthdays or achievements coming up. Plan if a short dinner, a gathering, or a quick FaceTime call is appropriate.
- **Monthly Habit:** Host or attend a "Success Sunday" or "Win Wednesday." For example, each month, gather a few friends or family members to share one win or highlight from their lives. This keeps everyone's spirits high and fosters deeper emotional connections.

Celebration Examples

- **Attend Their Event:** If someone close to you is celebrating a birthday or graduation, show up—even if it's for a short while. Presence matters.
- **Gift or Gesture:** If a friend landed a new job overseas, send them a small "bon voyage" package or plan a farewell meal.
- **Words of Affirmation:** Sometimes, a heartfelt letter, email, or a personal card is all it takes to make someone feel valued.

As a Boxing Life Coach, I see these activities as essential "social conditioning." Just as a fighter does roadwork to build stamina, we do "celebration work" to build relational stamina, ensuring our connections never run on empty.

Leverage: Tapping People, Resources, and Communities

You don't have to plan every celebration single-handedly. Like a champion boxer with a dedicated corner team, you can recruit help from multiple angles.

People:

- **Family & Close Friends:** Siblings, parents, and best friends might offer event-planning support or even host a celebration in their home.
- **Extended Community:** Gym buddies, church members, business colleagues. They can recommend venues or suggest ways to enrich the event (like games or group trips).

Resources:

- **Calendar Reminders:** Your phone's calendar can remind you of upcoming birthdays, anniversaries, or personal achievements (like "6-month mark at new job").
- **Online Platforms:**
    - **Amazon:** Perfect for quick gifts or special items to make the celebration memorable.
    - **Social Media Groups:** Whether it's a local meetup or a private Facebook or whatsapp group for close friends, these channels streamline coordination.

Communities:

- **Gym Circles:** If you're celebrating a fitness milestone—like finishing 72 days of Champ Camp—inviting gym friends can be powerful.
- **Church or Faith Communities:** If you're celebrating a spiritual milestone, or you want a venue for a wedding or baby dedication.
- **Neighborhood Associations:** Great if you're celebrating something that impacts local life, like finishing a community project or hosting a block party to reward team efforts.

Don't underestimate the synergy gained from collaborating. Just as a boxer needs a sparring partner to improve, you need your circle to make these celebrations lively and meaningful.

Score: Measuring Celebration Impact

It might sound odd to measure parties and gatherings, but reflection ensures you're making the most of these moments. Think of it like analyzing fight footage after a match—understanding what worked and what you can do better next time.

Lead KPIs (Actions You Control):

1. **Number of Celebrations Hosted or Attended:** Did you meet your monthly celebration goals?
2. **Invitations Sent:** Are you proactively including the crucial people in your life?
3. **Planning Consistency:** How often did you schedule a gathering or check in about upcoming milestones?

Lag KPIs (Results):

1. **Emotional Connection:** Do you feel closer to your family and friends? Have you noticed an increase in shared positivity or communal support?
2. **Feedback & Engagement:** Do your loved ones express gratitude for these celebrations? Are they reciprocating by inviting you to their events?
3. **Personal Fulfillment:** After each celebration, do you feel recharged, inspired, and more committed to your leadership role in the community?

Assess these metrics regularly. Maybe monthly or quarterly—whatever pace fits your lifestyle. If you find that you're hosting fewer events than intended or the emotional warmth is lacking, adjust your approach. Like a boxer tweaking a stance or guard, you refine your celebration tactics to yield stronger relational bonds and deeper satisfaction.

Personal Stories & Boxing Inspirations

I remember a moment when I coached a friend through a major life transition—he decided to move abroad to chase a bigger role in his company. After months of paperwork and emotional roller coasters, he finally boarded that plane. Instead of letting him slip away quietly, a group of us threw a heartfelt farewell gathering. We decorated a friend's living room with airplane motifs, gave mini speeches about our favorite memories with him, and shared a final group toast. The atmosphere was electric—laughter, tears, and a collective sense of triumph. That night anchored our friendships, and even across continents, we still connect via video calls with that nostalgic spark in our hearts.

Professional boxers often speak of the power of the final ring walk—the elaborate entrance that celebrates their persona and journey. Think of Tyson Fury's lively ring entrances or Floyd Mayweather's extravagant walkouts, complete with music, dancers, and celebrities. These spectacles aren't merely for show; they pump adrenaline into the fighter and unify fans in celebration. In a simpler way, each personal success we celebrate is our own "ring walk," a moment to say, "Yes, I've arrived at this milestone—now share it with me."

Building a Culture of Celebration

A consistent approach to celebrating success contributes to a culture where achievements are the norm, not the exception, and where unity thrives. People become more open about their aspirations, knowing that achievements will be met with genuine applause, not envy or apathy.

1. **Encourage Others to Celebrate:** When a friend lands a promotion, initiate a small gathering or at least a group dinner. They learn to pay it forward.

2. **Practice Gratitude Publicly:** In your circle, be the first to thank people out loud. "Thanks for always having my back, Mom and Dad," or "Without you guys, I'd never have finished this 72-day Champ Camp."
3. **Stay Humble While Embracing Joy:** Celebrations aren't about bragging; they're about community. A champion thanks the team and the fans, not just themselves.

By championing a culture of gratitude and celebration, you aren't just partying. You're uplifting the emotional tone of your circle, leading by example, and strengthening the bonds that make us all unstoppable.

A Call to Action: 12 Minutes to Plan Your Celebrations

It's time to apply the concepts from this chapter. Set aside 12 minutes for this activity:

1. **List 3-5 Major Milestones:** Look at the next 6-12 months. Are there birthdays, weddings, big moves, or challenges you or your loved ones are tackling? Jot them down.
2. **Brainstorm Up to 50 People:** Start with family, close friends, mentors, business partners, gym buddies—anyone who might be relevant to these milestones. Don't stress about hitting exactly 50, but aim for breadth.
3. **Apply the G.O.A.L.S. Framework:**

    - **Gratitude:** Who do you appreciate most within this list of 50? Write down names and why.
    - **Outcome:** Define your SMART plan for each milestone. Is it a small dinner, a weekend party, or an online get-together?
    - **Activities:** Outline how you'll celebrate: theme, location, personal touches.

- **Leverage:** Determine who'll help you plan and what resources you'll use.
- **Score:** Decide how you'll evaluate if the celebration strengthened relationships, boosted morale, and left a lasting positive vibe.

Document these ideas now. Trust me, the best celebrations are the ones that don't just "happen"—they're those you cultivate with care, like seeds in a garden.

Harnessing the Power of Community Joy

Celebrating success with family and friends is about more than just having fun. It's a strategic move that fosters gratitude, nurtures relationships, and multiplies everyone's motivation to keep striving. It's akin to a boxer's post-match press conference, where the fighter publicly acknowledges the trainer, the fans, and even the opponent—thus humanising the sport and reinforcing communal bonds.

By using the G.O.A.L.S. framework, you ensure these celebrations remain purposeful, not perfunctory. From planning (Gratitude, Outcome, Activities) to execution (Leverage) and reflection (Score), every step is a chance to do more than clink glasses. It's a chance to share your journey, pass on lessons, and light a fire in others.

In *A Year By Design*, celebrating success is the final step that binds all other efforts together. Whether you're generating £300,000 in turnover, publishing 33 books, conquering Champ Camp, or hitting the mainstream media, each achievement deserves a moment in the spotlight—shared with the people who matter most. So raise that metaphorical—or literal—championship belt, look your loved ones in the eye, and say, "We did it. Together."

That's what it means to celebrate like a champion.

13

Complete 72 Days of Champ Camp

Every champion's journey begins long before the lights come on, long before the roar of the crowd, and long before the ring announcer shouts their name. Behind every highlight reel is a secret world of sweat, pain, and uncompromising discipline—a regimen that tests a fighter's spirit as much as it tests their technique. That's the spirit I want to tap into with Champ Camp: an intensive, meticulously crafted approach to training like the greatest boxers in history. By dedicating 72 days out of the year to this system, we'll capture the essence of champion-level preparation and emerge stronger in body, mind, and soul.

As a Boxing Life Coach, I believe training isn't just about punishing your body until it aches. It's about forging mental resilience and unwavering confidence. It's about remembering that greatness is often decided in the lonely hours of early-morning roadwork or the final reps when your muscles are screaming to quit. The blueprint for this program draws from the training philosophies of legends such as Muhammad Ali, Floyd Mayweather Jr., Mike Tyson, Roy Jones Jr., and Manny Pacquiao. Additionally, I've gleaned insights from Gary Todd's *Greatest Boxing Workouts*—a treasure trove of real-life regimens employed by world champions—and from the thousands of hours I've spent studying fight documentaries, behind-the-scenes training footage, and cinematic portrayals of boxers.

This chapter is about unveiling Champ Camp, explaining how I plan to integrate it into my year, and, more importantly, challenging you to do the same. Let's lace up and step into the GOALS framework to take on the physical and mental gauntlet designed to transform us into the best versions of ourselves.

What is Champ Camp?

Champ Camp is a designated period of boxing-inspired training, spread out over the year. My aim: **72 days** of intense, champion-like workouts. Rather than 72 consecutive days, I'll distribute these sessions to fit my schedule: I will dedicate 5 x 3 week mini camps, one dedicated to each. This approach yields well over 72 sessions—closer to 90—but I'm committing to hitting at least 72 in total. Why 72? Because it's both realistic and challenging enough to demand everything I've got.

A single Champ Camp day includes:

- **A Cardio Block:** Typically a 5-16 km run or similar steady-state cardio.
- **A Boxing Session:** Focus on technique, bag work, pad work, and intense punching drills (3,000-5,000 punches in total).
- **A Strength & Conditioning Slot:** Could be sprints, plyometrics, or calisthenics that push endurance, speed and raw power.

By the end of each day, we aim to log a "10k+ deposit" into our training bank—meaning a combination of running and punches (or reps) that hits at least 10,000 total movements. It's an aggressive target, reminiscent of the champion mindsets we admire.

G.O.A.L.S. Framework

We'll apply the five-step G.O.A.L.S. framework, just like in previous chapters:

1. **Gratitude**
2. **Outcome**
3. **Activities**
4. **Leverage**
5. **Score**

Let's break it all down.

Gratitude: Acknowledge What Already Enables Our Success

Whenever a fighter claims a title, they thank their corner, their coaches, and often a higher power for the journey. Before we dive into Champ Camp, let's center ourselves in appreciation for the gifts and resources that make it possible.

Five Things I'm Grateful For

1. **My Love for Boxing:** I'm not forcing myself to train; I genuinely enjoy the sport's nuances and the thrill of pushing my physical limits.
2. **My Youth & Health:** At this stage of my life, my body is capable of handling rigorous activity, and I have minimal injuries.
3. **High-Quality Mentorship from the Greats:** Although I haven't trained directly with Ali or Tyson, their philosophies and stories serve as mental and tactical guides.
4. **Previous Intense Training Experience:** I've completed high-intensity regimens before, so my body and mind know how to handle the stress.
5. **Shared Inspiration & Community:** I'm surrounded by driven people—trainers, friends, fans—who ignite my motivation to keep punching, running, and innovating.

Muhammad Ali once said, "It's the repetition of affirmations that leads to belief. And once that belief becomes a deep conviction, things begin to happen." My gratitude statements are my affirmations, reminding me why this journey is worth undertaking.

Outcome: Defining Our Goal with Precision
SMART Goal:
I will **complete 72 days of Champ Camp** by December 31, 2025, each day consisting of a fundamental boxing training routine for mental focus, confidence, and resilience. My plan is to do 3 weeks for each of the 5 champions I have been studying, ensuring I surpass 72 sessions comfortably.

Why It Matters: Key Checkpoints & Motivations

- **Checkpoints:**

    1. **18 Days Completed** – The first big chunk, a psychological victory.
    2. **36 Days Completed** – Halfway point, a testament to consistency.
    3. **54 Days Completed** – Nearing the finish line, motivation intensifies.
    4. **72 Days Completed** – Mission accomplished.
- **My Why—Top Ten Reasons for Champ Camp**

    1. **Inspiring Others to Get Back in Shape:** By sharing my journey, I hope to show people what disciplined boxing can do for health and confidence.
    2. **Staying Ready for Boxing Opportunities:** If a chance to compete or spar arises, I'll be physically primed.
    3. **Achieving My Best Physical Condition:** Push past current limits, forging next-level strength and endurance.
    4. **Surrounded by Great Fighters:** Being in an environment of top-level fighters—past and present—fuels my drive.

5. **Improving Overall Health:** A robust training regimen wards off stress, boosts cardiovascular health, and lifts mental well-being.
6. **Developing My Boxing Abilities:** Refining footwork, timing, and power, taking technical cues from Ali's footwork to Tyson's devastating hooks.
7. **Reaching Fighting Weight (Welterweight):** A structured plan to maintain or cut weight responsibly.
8. **Mastery to Coach Others:** Learning from intense training helps me guide clients through their own programs.
9. **Mental & Physical Test:** Challenges like these reveal and refine character, ensuring I carry resilience into every area of life.
10. **Setting a Positive Example:** For family, friends, and community. I want them to see grit in action, not just hear talk.

This approach turns a vague dream ("train like a pro fighter") into a measurable reality. As Manny Pacquiao notes, "Discipline is the bridge between your boxing goals and your boxing accomplishments." Precisely. Our outcome is defined, and the path is set.

Activities: Breaking Down the Training Routine

Champ Camp isn't a casual "gym day." It's a rigorous, structured plan that demands consistency. We'll integrate three main components—**Cardio**, **Boxing**, and **Conditioning**—in 2-3 sessions per day.

Typical Day Breakdown

1. **Cardio (5 km – 16 km)**

    ◦ **Morning Run:** Start with 5-16 kilometers, depending on your current stamina or training focus. On heavier days, you might push closer to 16 km at a steady pace; on lighter days, 5 km of intervals or sprints might suffice.

2. **Boxing Session (Second Session)**

    - **Technique & Punch Count:** Aim for 3,000 to 5,000 punches—mix jabs, crosses, hooks, uppercuts. Incorporate shadowboxing, heavy bag, pad work, and speed bag.
    - **Drills from Gary Todd's Book:** Todd's *Greatest Boxing Workouts* compiles champion routines. For instance, Mayweather's approach to pad work or Mike Tyson's peek-a-boo style can be adapted for your skill level.
    - **Rounds & Intensity:** Typically, 10-36 rounds on the shadowboxing, on the bag, hitting the pads or shadowboxing, each lasting 3-4 minutes, with 30-60 second rests.

3. **Strength & Conditioning (Third Session)**

    - **Sprints or Plyometrics:** A short, intense sprint session or jump squats for explosive power, reminiscent of Manny Pacquiao's hill sprints in the Filipino mountains.
    - **Calisthenics/Circuit Training:** Push-ups, pull-ups, burpees, medicine ball throws, or kettlebell swings. Roy Jones Jr. championed bodyweight circuits that kept him agile and powerful.
    - **Core & Flexibility:** Planks, medicine ball twists, or yoga-like stretches to maintain fluid movement in the ring.

Scheduling Across the Year

- **Three Weeks of Each Fighter (5 times):** Monday through Saturday intensives, adding up to extra sessions.
- **Second Half of 2025:** Another high-intensity day to keep the routine from getting stale.

With 18 days for each inspiring champion, you'll surpass 72 days in total—likely hitting around 90. This way, even if you miss a day or two due to illness or scheduling, you can still comfortably meet the 72-day target.

Leverage: Tapping into Inspiration, People, and Resources

No boxer fights alone. Even "one-man show" personas like Floyd Mayweather had essential support—a father who was once a pro fighter, an uncle who guided his defensive strategy, and a stable of sparring partners.

People & Inspirations

- **Past Champions (Muhammad Ali, Floyd Mayweather, Roy Jones Jr., Manny Pacquiao, Mike Tyson):** Their documented training methods, interviews, and fights are goldmines of motivation.
- **Present Champions (Canelo Alvarez, Naoya Inoue, Terence Crawford, Oleksandr Usyk, Gervonta Davis):** Observing today's best keeps you updated on modern training techniques and strategy evolutions.
- **Local Boxing Gym & Coaching Staff:** Engage with a coach who can spot weaknesses in your form, provide real-time feedback, and hold you accountable.

Resources

- **YouTube & Documentaries:** Hours of behind-the-scenes footage featuring the likes of Ali's roadwork at 5 a.m., Manny Pacquiao's intense pad sessions with Freddie Roach, or Tyson's savage bag drills in Catskill, New York.

- **Gary Todd's** *Greatest Boxing Workouts*: The official text for champion-level insights. Study it, highlight tips, and adapt them to your skill level.
- **Equipment & Environments:** A quality pair of gloves, good running shoes, a heavy bag, jump rope, plus open spaces like local parks or running tracks.

Communities

- **Boxing Gym or Health Club:** Join a local boxing gym or even a typical fitness centre that has boxing equipment. You'll find training partners, potential sparring mates, and coaches.
- **Running Clubs:** They can help keep your cardio on point. Even Mayweather would sometimes run with a group to push pace.
- **Online Forums or Facebook Groups:** For accountability and tips—some groups focus on specific boxing challenges, sharing daily progress, or exchanging training videos.

Ali said, "I'm so fast that last night I turned off the light switch in my hotel room and was in bed before the room was dark." Humour aside, his confidence and flair came from leveraging top-quality trainers, supportive communities, and unyielding self-belief. We replicate that approach by leaning on proven resources.

Score: Measuring Your Champ Camp Progress

We don't want to punch blindly in the dark. Like a fighter who diligently counts combos, times miles, or tracks heart rates, we must quantify progress.

Key Performance Indicators (KPIs)

- **Lead KPIs (Actions You Control)**

1. **Number of Champ Camp Days Attended:** Log each Champ Camp day completed.
2. **Punch Count per Session:** Aim for 10-36 rounds of boxing. With an average of 200 punches a round, it will be 2,000 to 7,200 punches, or at least record approximate tallies. This metric ensures your form and endurance keep growing.
3. **Running Distance/Terrain Type:** Track whether you ran 5 km or 16 km, if it was intervals or steady. Variation fosters a well-rounded cardio base.

- **Lag KPIs (Outcome Indicators)**

1. **Completion of 72 Sessions:** The grand milestone, the final bell signifying your victory.
2. **Weight & Body Composition:** If you aim to reach welterweight, measure weight or body-fat percentage monthly to ensure you're trending in the right direction.
3. **Skill and Confidence Growth:** This is qualitative—do you feel more fluid in the ring? Are your sparring partners noticing sharper technique?

Measuring Frequency

- **Weekly Check-Ins:** Confirm you completed Champ Camp sessions for the week. If not, can you reschedule?
- **Monthly Evaluations:** Tally how many sessions you did and whether you adhered to the "10k+ deposit" target. Reassess your punch forms, cardio times, or weight.
- **Quarterly Reflection:** Each quarter (end of that "Champ Camp week"), see if you hit your day count. Evaluate if you're pacing well toward 72 total sessions.

Celebrating Wins

- **18, 36, 54, 72 Days:** Each checkpoint is a small championship in itself. Treat yourself—maybe a boxing gear upgrade at 18 days, a spa session at 36, new shoes at 54, and a serious celebratory dinner at 72.
- **Mentor Feedback:** At major checkpoints, share your progress with a coach or training partner for external validation and advice.

Personal Stories: The Drive Behind the Routine

I remember a phase in my life when I was enthralled by Floyd Mayweather Jr.'s midnight training. Stories emerged of him hitting the gym at 2 a.m., or going for a road run at 3 a.m., while the rest of the world slept. Initially, it sounded insane. But the more I studied him, the more I understood: success in the ring wasn't just about a fight night game plan—it was about outworking the competition when nobody else was looking.

Likewise, Manny Pacquiao's famed hill sprints in the Philippines highlight the ethic of a champion whose heart is as big as his skill set. Roy Jones Jr. might run with chickens in rural Florida—like in that iconic scene capturing his speed and agility. Or consider how Mike Tyson hammered out thousands of sit-ups daily, forging iron-like abs for rib-breaking body shots. These anecdotes revealed a consistent theme: champion-level achievements demand champion-level training.

At times, I've tried to emulate aspects of these routines, picking and choosing bits of Ali's swagger, Pacquiao's sprints, or Tyson's calisthenics. Each experiment taught me something new about grit, mental discipline, and how the body can adapt to extraordinary demands if the mind remains resolute. Now, by formalising that approach into Champ Camp, I'm giving shape to a personal legacy of discipline—one that I hope resonates with my clients, fans, and loved ones, showing them that with the right blueprint, they too can transform.

The Power of Testing Limits

Boxing is more than jabs and hooks—it's a metaphor for resilience, courage, and strategic thinking. If you can endure a 2-4 hour training day that packs in running, bag work, pad sessions, and conditioning, you can endure a demanding project at work, an emotionally draining family crisis, or the rigors of pursuing big business goals. Each day of Champ Camp is like forging mental steel: you face your own fatigue, your own doubts, and prove that neither can stop you.

Mike Tyson said, "Everybody has a plan until they get punched in the mouth." Champ Camp is about forging a plan that can endure life's inevitable "punches." Maybe you'll face unexpected work deadlines, family emergencies, or injuries. The discipline you gain from repeated intense sessions arms you with the mental toughness to adapt gracefully without abandoning your goals.

A Culture of Excellence

Engaging in a structured program also helps those around you. If you're consistent with Monday workouts or you're devoting the first week of each quarter to hardcore training, people around you notice. They see your hustle, your discipline, and your unwavering commitment. This can spark conversations like, "What are you doing differently?" or "How do you find the motivation?" This is where your role as a Boxing Life Coach expands beyond yourself—you become a living billboard of resilience, inspiring others to push their boundaries.

A Call to Action: Plan Your Own Champ Camp in 12 Minutes

I invite you to spend the next 12 minutes drafting your personal Champ Camp blueprint:

1. **Define Your Session Count & Schedule:**

- How many days will you commit to? 30? 50? Go bold—72 or 100 if you dare.
- Which days fit your calendar best? Maybe every Sunday, or a block of days each month?

2. **Map Your Training Blocks:**

    - **Cardio:** Decide running distances or times. Intervals or steady state?
    - **Boxing Technique:** Bag work, shadowboxing, combos, or specialized drills.
    - **Conditioning:** Sprints, calisthenics, or plyometric circuits.
    - **Champion Inspirations:** Will you follow more of a Tyson approach (power) or a Mayweather approach (stamina, defense)?

3. **Leverage Your Circle:**

    - Who can keep you accountable?
    - Which gym or running club can you join?
    - How do you incorporate your schedule, perhaps using apps like Strava or MyFitnessPal?

4. **Track & Celebrate:**

    - Create a chart or note on your phone to mark each Champ Camp day completed.
    - Decide small or big treats at intermediate milestones—maybe new gloves at half the target, a short getaway at the end.

Write it down. Commit to a number. If you're serious, you'll find the time to push yourself, forging a champion's mindset in every corner of your life.

Stepping Into the Ring of Self-Mastery

Completing 72 days of Champ Camp is more than a fitness journey. It's a testament to your capability to design a year that merges ambition, discipline, and self-belief. Like Floyd Mayweather once said, "Hard work, dedication"—that's the formula. By structuring your workouts, gleaning inspiration from legendary fighters, and relentlessly testing your body, you transform from "aspiring doer" to "active champion."

When you endure the 5 a.m. run, the relentless round on the bag, the sets of sprints that leave your legs shaking, you're not just training your body—you're training your spirit. Each punch thrown or kilometer run is a deposit in the bank of your resilience. And with every deposit, you become more and more unstoppable, both inside and outside the ring.

In *A Year By Design*, your champ-level training isn't a random footnote. It's a core element that shapes your identity as a Boss, Fighter, Champion, Man of God, Boxing Life Coach, Super Author, Lover, and Family Man. Because if you can master your body and willpower in this way, you'll channel that mastery into every other role you hold, achieving breakthroughs that leave onlookers wondering how you do it all.

So, lace up the gloves. Warm up that engine with a 5-kilometer run. Let the heart pound and the sweat flow. Focus on the daily discipline needed to inch toward 72 (or more) days of champion-inspired training. One day, you'll look back—maybe at day 73—and realise you've become the kind of fighter in life that even your past idols would applaud. That's the essence of Champ Camp: forging a champion's heart to tackle everything life throws at you.

Welcome to the ring. It's time to train like you mean it.

14

Train Like a Fighter for 300 Days

There's a certain feeling you get when you lace up gloves and step into a ring, even if you're just training and not competing. It's a unique tension—equal parts fear, excitement, and purpose. You can feel your heart pounding in your ears while your mind sharpens, ready to execute every jab, cross, or hook you've drilled into muscle memory. Over countless hours, this intense dedication transforms your body and hardens your mindset.

This chapter isn't about fight-night glory. It's about the daily grind that molds ordinary people into fighters, forging discipline, grit, and physical excellence. We'll explore how to *train like a fighter for 300 days*, weaving daily workouts into the fabric of your routine so that you, too, can taste the transformative power of consistent, high-level boxing-inspired training. If you've ever wondered how fighters like Muhammad Ali, Floyd Mayweather Jr., Mike Tyson, Roy Jones Jr., and Manny Pacquiao built unstoppable engines, you're about to see how their principles can shape your life.

I'm inviting you to set aside 300 days of training—just 45 minutes a day, minimum. By the end of those 300 days, you won't just have a stronger body; you'll have a sharper mind, a more resilient spirit, and a renewed sense of what's possible when you challenge yourself to think and move like a fighter.

What Does It Mean to Train Like a Fighter?
Let's clarify the concept:

1. **Daily Commitment:** You devote at least 45 minutes each day to structured training—no excuses.
2. **Core Components:** Each session includes **cardio** (running/sprints), **combat training** (bag work, shadowboxing, jump rope, padwork, sparring if available), and/or **conditioning** (circuit exercises, core workouts, bodyweight drills).
3. **Quarterly R&R:** After each quarter (roughly every three months), you'll take a short break—a week off or reduced-volume training—to recover, reflect, and come back fresher.

Boxers fuse these elements to prepare for the ring. In the same vein, you'll harness them to reach peak fitness, mental toughness, and possibly learn basic self-defense along the way. As legendary trainer Cus D'Amato once said, "The hero and the coward feel the same fear, but the hero uses his fear and projects it onto his opponent." Our aim is to channel our daily stresses and uncertainties into a constructive force that shapes us for the better.

G.O.A.L.S. Framework

Like previous chapters, we'll apply the five-part G.O.A.L.S. framework:

1. **Gratitude**
2. **Outcome**
3. **Activities**
4. **Leverage**
5. **Score**

This ensures we don't just talk about training—we integrate it intentionally, much like designing any other major life goal.

Gratitude: Acknowledging the Tools and Blessings That Empower Us

Before we dive into the daily grind, let's highlight what already sets us up for success. Gratitude anchors us, reminding us that training isn't just a chore or punishment; it's an opportunity.

Five (or More) Things I'm Grateful For

1. **I've Done It Before:** I've already pushed my body and mind to similar extremes, whether for amateur boxing or K1 competitions. Past experience is a springboard to go even further.
2. **Competitive Background:** Having stepped into the ring, I understand the discipline needed, and that inside knowledge is a precious gift many people never experience.
3. **A Deep Love for Boxing:** It's not just a means to sweat—I genuinely enjoy the sport's technique, culture, and history. Passion acts as rocket fuel for perseverance.
4. **Scheduled Recovery:** Knowing I get a few days off a year (especially that quarterly break) prevents burnout. Short rests are crucial.
5. **Natural Fighting Instinct:** God blessed me with decent reflexes and hand-eye coordination. For me, fighting truly does feel like second nature.
6. **Elevating My Brand:** As a Boxing Life Coach, living what I preach builds authenticity. When people see the shape I maintain, they trust my guidance more.

Muhammad Ali said, "It's the repetition of affirmations that leads to belief." Repetitions of gratitude reinforce the mindset that you have everything you need to succeed—no matter the obstacles.

Outcome: Defining a Fighter's Training Goal

A champion doesn't just float through workouts; they set targets. For you, it's **300 days** of training that merges cardio, combat, and conditioning. Simple enough, right?

SMART Format

- **Specific:** "I will train like a fighter for 300 days within one calendar year, dedicating at least 45 minutes each day to cardio, combat training, and conditioning."
- **Measurable:** 300 training sessions ticked off in a log or phone app. You can't cheat the numbers.
- **Achievable:** 45 minutes a day is doable for most lifestyles—carve out early mornings, lunch breaks, or evenings.
- **Relevant:** If your goals include better fitness, a sharper mind, improved discipline, or just an everyday hero's stamina, this is perfect.
- **Time-Bound:** A one-year horizon gives structure, with breaks each quarter to keep you fresh and motivated.

Checkpoints

1. **30 Days:** Enough to notice improvements in stamina, mental clarity, and overall energy.
2. **100 Days:** A massive chunk—where old habits are replaced, and you start feeling like an athlete.
3. **150 Days:** The halfway point. Endurance, power, and confidence are peaking.
4. **200 Days:** Smoother technique, possibly a new personal record in running or a more fluid punch combination.
5. **300 Days:** Mission accomplished—a fighter's discipline etched into your daily routine.

Why This Matters: Top Ten Reasons to Train Like a Fighter for 300 Days

1. **Peak Physical Fitness:** Explosive power, endurance, agility, balance—boxers are multi-faceted athletes, and this regimen sculpts your body to perform on all fronts.
2. **Mental Toughness:** Overcoming daily discomfort fosters resilience, filtering into every aspect of life—business, relationships, personal challenges.
3. **Consistent Progress:** 300 days forces you to adopt routines—healthy eating, structured exercise, and mindful recovery. The compounding effect is transformative.
4. **Weight & Body Composition:** High-intensity training melts fat, builds muscle, and encourages sustainable weight management.
5. **Confidence Building:** Acquiring punching skills and defending techniques changes your posture and aura. People sense your newfound solidity.
6. **Stress Relief & Emotional Balance:** Boxing combos, sprints, and circuit drills serve as daily therapy, releasing endorphins that stabilize emotions.
7. **Structured Routine:** A set schedule fosters discipline—essential for success in all domains.
8. **Self-Defense Skills:** You're not just hitting a bag; you're mastering practical movements that could protect you if needed.
9. **Community & Accountability:** Boxing rarely happens in isolation—gyms, clubs, or training partners become your supportive cast.
10. **Leadership by Example:** Friends and family see your dedication, often adopting healthier habits themselves.

What Happens If You Don't Train Like a Fighter

1. **Slower Physical Progress:** Sporadic workouts yield lukewarm results, leaving you disappointed or plateaued.
2. **Weaker Mental Fortitude:** A fighter's regimen pushes you mentally. Skipping it means missing out on a crucible that builds self-trust and resilience.
3. **Inconsistent Lifestyle Habits:** Without the daily anchor of training, nutritional and recovery practices can slip, scattering your focus.
4. **Higher Stress Levels:** The explosive outlet that punching a bag or sprinting provides might be absent, risking pent-up tension and anxiety.
5. **Reduced Accountability:** Without a structured plan, your circle of gym buddies or coaches can't effectively keep you on track, leading to drifting fitness goals.

Activities: Daily, Weekly, and Monthly Habits for a Fighter's Routine

If "Train Like a Fighter" is our mantra, then each day we must enact the ritual. My recommendation: **at least 45 minutes** of dedicated training that combines three core elements—**cardio, combat training**, and **conditioning**.

Daily Structure

1. **Cardio (Running/Sprints)**

   - Aim for a **5 km run** at a moderate pace. If 5 km feels too easy, consider intervals or longer distances.
   - Alternative: Hills or sprint circuits, especially if you're short on time but want high intensity.

2. **Combat Training**

    - **Shadowboxing (3-5 rounds):** Refine footwork and hand speed. Visualise an opponent; practice defensive moves.
    - **Bag Work (3-5 rounds):** Prioritise technique—jabs, hooks, uppercuts. Manny Pacquiao hammered the heavy bag daily for power.
    - **Pad Work or Sparring (if available):** Floyd Mayweather's famous pad routines help refine timing and precision. If you have a partner, nothing beats live feedback.
    - **Jump Rope (3 rounds of 2-3 minutes):** Boost footwork and stamina. Roy Jones Jr. credited rope skipping for his legendary agility.

3. **Conditioning**

    - **Bodyweight Circuits:** Push-ups, burpees, squats, lunges, planks, core drills. Mike Tyson reportedly did up to 2,000 sit-ups a day in his prime. Manny Pacquiao too.
    - **Resistance Training:** Kettlebells, resistance bands, medicine balls, or light free weights to build explosive power.
    - **Stretching & Mobility:** Prevent injuries and enhance movement range, essential for fluid boxing.

Weekly Rhythm

- **Monday-Tuesday:** Combine run + 2-3 hour gym session if time permits. These early-week sessions set the tone.
- **Wednesday:** 5 km run or lighter day focusing on technique.
- **Thursday:** Another 2-hour gym block, focusing on skill refinement and heavier conditioning.

- **Friday:** 5 km run + technical training—perhaps focusing on combos or footwork.
- **Saturday:** 2-3 hours intense session—think "Champ Camp Lite," or add sparring if an opportunity arises.
- **Sunday:** Active recovery—a 5 km walk or light jog, plus optional sparring or skills-based practice.

Monthly and Quarterly Adjustments

- **Every Month:** Evaluate your progress. Are you handling 5 km easily? Bump it to 7 km or try intervals. Are you bored with the same combos? Integrate new drills from videos or books.
- **Quarterly Break:** After 3 months of consistent training, allow yourself a week off or a heavily reduced schedule. This rest & recovery helps avoid burnout and muscle overuse.

This daily blueprint fosters a boxer's endurance and skill without forcing you to live at the gym. The consistent 45-minute minimum secures progress, while optional extended sessions accelerate your results.

Leverage: People, Resources, and Communities to Elevate Your Game

Boxers don't walk into the ring alone. They rely on corners, cutmen, coaches, and a robust support system. Your quest is no different.

People

1. **Jonathan Reid (Accountability Partner):** He checks in weekly, ensuring I never miss the daily 45-minute session and that I keep my schedule balanced.
2. **Ultimate Masterclasses Coaching Systems:** Possibly a selection of specialised trainers that manage training cycles and diet suggestions.

3. **Clients & Friends:** Let them see your progress. Let them challenge you. When you have eyes on your journey, you'll push harder.

Resources

1. **Training Videos on YouTube:** Documentaries or short clips showing how Ali ran, how Mayweather hit pads, or how Manny hammered the bag.
2. **Books (e.g., *Greatest Boxing Workouts*):** Another deep well of ideas. Cross-reference the workouts of champion fighters to keep your regimen fresh.
3. **Apple Watch or Fitness Tracker:** Monitor heart rate, track distances, and record daily activity for data-driven accountability.

Community

1. **David Lloyd Gyms:** Known for quality facilities—access to well-equipped boxing areas, classes, or personal trainers.
2. **Key Results Club:** A dedicated group focusing on personal development. If they emphasize fitness, you can find synergy here.
3. **Nike Run Club, Park Run & Run with Re:** Perfect for the running segment. Virtual run clubs or local chapters can keep your cardio honest.
4. **Define Fitness, London Martial Arts Academy and other boxing gyms:** If you're near these gyms, they could be your daily training ground, offering classes, sparring sessions, or just a communal environment.

Leaning on these resources ensures you're not left to do guesswork or lose motivation. Tyson Fury once said, "A champion must train in Hell to live in Heaven." This might be an overstatement, but with the right support network, training feels less like Hell and more like a thrilling path to glory.

Score: Measuring Training Impact Over 300 Days

A fighter meticulously logs rounds, punch counts, and sparring performance. We do the same, but at a holistic level.

Lead KPIs

1. **Days Completed:** Maintain a simple chart or phone note to tick off each day you fulfill the 45-minute minimum. You're aiming for 300 ticks by year's end.
2. **Distance Run & Punch Volume:** Record how many kilometers you run and how many rounds boxed (approximate). Variation fosters improvement.
3. **Workout Diversity:** Track if you're including conditioning and skill-based work. The right mix keeps your training well-rounded.

Lag KPIs

1. **Major Checkpoints:** 30 days, 100 days, 150 days, 200 days, and 300 days. Celebrate each milestone to sustain excitement.
2. **Physical Changes:** Weight, body fat, muscular definition. Are you dropping weight or adding lean muscle? Evaluate monthly or quarterly.
3. **Skill Progress:** Can you last more rounds on the bag without losing form? Is your footwork sharper during sparring?

Celebration & Reflection

- **At Each Checkpoint:** Reward yourself—maybe new boxing gloves at day 100, a mini-vacation at day 200, a big feast at day 300.

- **Quarterly Review:** Inspect your logs. If you missed more days than expected, realign your schedule or ask your accountability partner to hold you tighter to your goals.

Personal Anecdotes & Lessons from Legendary Fighters

1. **Muhammad Ali's Roadwork:** Known to run at dawn while reciting self-affirmations like "I'm the greatest." He used these silent hours to mentally train as well.
2. **Mike Tyson's 4 a.m. Runs:** D'Amato insisted on early runs to mentally get ahead of any opponent. Tyson often said, "If I do it while they're asleep, I'm working harder than them."
3. **Manny Pacquiao's Hill Sprints:** Pacquiao's stamina is the stuff of legends. Observing his hill runs reveals unmatched determination. Sparring 36 rounds before a fight.
4. **Floyd Mayweather's Late-Night Gym Sessions:** He'd head to the gym in the early hours, believing it gave him an edge. "Hard work, dedication" might be clichéd, but it fueled Floyd's undefeated record.
5. **Roy Jones Jr.'s Creative Training:** Known for unorthodox methods—he even played basketball on the same day as a fight to keep agile and to test his abilities. It underscores how variety can keep training fresh and dynamic.

These anecdotes aren't meant to turn you into a professional fighter. They're examples of the extremes champions go to, inspiring you to find your own threshold for consistency, discipline, and innovation.

The 12 Key Principles of Success

Training like a fighter aligns with the *12 key principles of success* we've touched on in *A Year By Design*. Let's see how:

1. **Faith:** Believing in your ability to sustain daily training.
2. **Vision:** Envisioning the stronger, faster you at day 300.
3. **Teamwork:** Mentors, training partners, and supportive communities fuel your journey.
4. **Focus:** 45 minutes a day, no distractions—pure concentration on form and effort.
5. **Hard Work & Dedication:** No shortcuts. Boxing demands sincerity in every jab or sprint.
6. **Discipline:** On days you don't feel like training, you show up anyway. That's discipline.
7. **Will to Win:** A fighter's heart is tested daily. You keep going because that flame inside you says, "I'm not done yet."
8. **Resilience:** Physical exhaustion, plateaus—these are the lumps a fighter learns to roll with.
9. **Confidence:** Each completed workout injects self-belief. Confidence radiates outward into your everyday life.
10. **Respect:** Respect your body's limits, your trainers, and the centuries-old craft of boxing.
11. **Humility:** A single tough sparring session can remind you there's always more to learn.
12. **Legacy:** Whether you compete or not, you're leaving a personal legacy of determination that others will note and admire.

A Call to Action: 12 Minutes to Shape Your Fighter's Journey

Ready to commit? Grab a timer and invest **12 minutes** to draft your own "Train Like a Fighter for 300 Days" blueprint.

1. **Define Your 300-Day Timeline:** Are you starting immediately? Which months or weeks might be more challenging (holidays, busy seasons)?
2. **Outline Your Daily Routine:** Minimum 45 minutes. Decide the ratio of cardio, combat, and conditioning.

3. **Select Accountability Partners:** Could be a friend, a local boxing gym, or an online forum.
4. **Identify Inspirational Figures & Resources:** Any docuseries or fight highlight reels you'll turn to when motivation dips? Add them to a watchlist.
5. **Create a Log System:** Paper chart or phone note? How often will you update it?
6. **Plan Rewards:** You might gift yourself new gear at the halfway mark or a short holiday after day 300.

By the time the timer beeps, you'll have a rough outline of your journey. Then, it's a matter of daily, consistent execution. Like stepping into round one of a fight, the real test of heart begins.

Becoming the Fighter in Your Own Story

Training like a fighter for 300 days is more than a fitness goal; it's a statement about who you are and who you aim to become. You're deciding that complacency isn't an option, that you value mental and physical excellence, and that you refuse to settle for half-measures. Each day, each run, each set of punches on the heavy bag, represents another rung on the ladder of your potential.

Mike Tyson famously said, "Discipline is doing what you hate to do but doing it like you love it." Whether you love or hate the burn of a 5 km run, the sting of bag work, or the sweat from conditioning drills, you'll learn to *love* the result— a sharper mind, a stronger body, and a champion's spirit that radiates into everything you do. In your career, relationships, or community involvement, this unstoppable mindset will set you apart.

So, slip on those gloves. Lace up the running shoes. Plan your daily 45 minutes. Decide how you'll push through the next 300 days. Once you emerge on the other side, panting and proud, you'll have lived a slice of the fighter's life. And trust me, it's a life that redefines what you believe you can conquer. You become the champion of your own story, forging an iron will that thrives in the ring of life.

15

Think Like a Champion for 300 Days

Champions are made long before they ever appear in the spotlight. In the world of boxing, it's easy to focus on fight night, bright lights, and roaring crowds. Yet, the real magic unfolds away from the arena—early morning runs, rigorous mental drills, and unwavering self-belief cultivated day in and day out. That's the essence of **"thinking like a champion."** You train your mind to see hurdles as opportunities, setbacks as lessons, and the daily grind as the stepping stone to something remarkable.

In this chapter, we will explore what it means to think like a champion for 300 days. Rather than letting doubt and negativity seep into your routine, you'll practice the mental discipline that legendary fighters—Muhammad Ali, Floyd Mayweather Jr., Mike Tyson, Roy Jones Jr., and Manny Pacquiao—embodied in their careers. We'll connect it to the physical dimension—your daily 5 km+ run, your bagwork and pad sessions, your stretching, and your floor work. Because to me, *thinking* like a champion isn't just sitting still and visualizing success; it's a synergy between mind and body, confidence and sweat, clarity and action.

By the end of these 300 days, you won't just be in better shape physically—you'll have ingrained a resilient, optimistic, and tenacious mindset that can catapult you toward your goals in every corner of life.

Why "Think Like a Champion"?

Before we jump into the G.O.A.L.S. framework, let's define our terms. **"Thinking like a champion"** is about:

- **Harnessing inner dialogue to fuel performance:** Champions push through adversity by believing they can—and will—overcome any obstacle.
- **Reframing failures and setbacks:** Champions see losses as lessons. Instead of worrying about setbacks, they pivot, learn, and come back stronger.
- **Committing to daily mental practice:** Much like physical conditioning, mental conditioning is repeated until it feels second nature.

Ali once said, "Champions aren't made in gyms. Champions are made from something they have deep inside them—**a desire, a dream, a vision.**" That's what we're nurturing here: the desire, dream, and vision that keep us on track day after day.

The G.O.A.L.S. Framework

As with earlier chapters, we use the five-part G.O.A.L.S. framework—**Gratitude, Outcome, Activities, Leverage, Score**—to ensure we systematically incorporate champion-like thinking into our daily lives.

1. **Gratitude**
2. **Outcome**
3. **Activities**
4. **Leverage**
5. **Score**

Gratitude: Appreciating the Foundation for Success

Before we embark on any grand challenge, it's crucial to remember what blessings and resources we already have. This sense of gratitude keeps us grounded, optimistic, and aware that the road ahead is navigable precisely because of the support and gifts in our corner.

Five (or More) Things I'm Grateful For

1. **I've Done It Before**
   I've competed in amateur boxing and K1 competitions, so I know the highs, lows, and mental demands of combat sports. This prior exposure is a big advantage—I'm not starting from zero.

2. **My Love for Boxing**
   This isn't just about training. I genuinely admire the craft, the technique, and the discipline boxing requires. My passion makes the journey far more rewarding.

3. **Natural Fighting Instinct**
   Fighting and moving athletically come more naturally to me than to many others. Recognizing that grace is something I never want to take for granted.

4. **Scheduled Days Off**
   The idea that I can take a few days off every quarter—while still fulfilling the bigger picture—is liberating. Champions know the value of strategic rest.

5. **Better Shape, Better Brand**
   Improving my mental fortitude adds direct value to my brand as a Boxing Life Coach. People believe in what they see you live out.

While gratitude sets the tone for positivity, it also acts like a moral anchor—reminding me that I'm not alone, and that many of the resources I need are already at my fingertips. Legendary fighters often credited their trainers, families, or even God for their success, highlighting the same principle: behind every champion's mental toughness lies a bedrock of support and advantage.

Outcome: Setting a Clear, Measurable Goal

We're not here to dabble. We're here to **think like a champion for 300 days**—that means structuring a daily practice that ensures mental discipline is as integral to our routine as brushing our teeth. Let's define it with the SMART approach.

SMART Goal

- **Specific:** "I will invest a minimum of **20 minutes** each day for 300 days in dedicated champion mindset exercises—visualisation, affirmations, reading, or structured mental drills—while also aligning my daily physical training to reinforce this mindset."
- **Measurable:** I'll keep track of each day completed in a log or app, marking 300 successful mental-training days by year's end.
- **Achievable:** 20 minutes is modest but potent. The synergy with a 5 km+ run or boxing session ensures the mind-body connection is front and center.
- **Relevant:** A champion's mindset translates to better performance in the ring, at work, in relationships, and in life. It fortifies discipline, resilience, and leadership skills.
- **Time-Bound:** Over the course of a calendar year, with a week off each quarter, making sure to maintain the routine even around those rest periods.

Checkpoints

1. **30 Days:** Enough time to see your mental outlook begin to shift—less negativity, more self-assurance.
2. **100 Days:** A significant milestone where daily practice is almost second nature.
3. **150 Days:** By now, champion-level thinking might color how you handle adversity—failures or setbacks no longer rattle you as before.

4. **200 Days:** Confidence soars, and you may notice improvements across personal and professional realms.
5. **300 Days:** Mission accomplished. You've spent most of the year refining mental toughness, setting the stage for a lifetime of success.

Why It Matters: Top Ten Reasons to Think Like a Champion for 300 Days

1. **Consistent Motivation**
   A champion's mindset ensures you push through everyday challenges without burning out.
2. **Greater Resilience**
   Reframing failures as lessons fosters quicker comebacks from setbacks.
3. **Heightened Focus & Productivity**
   Mental discipline kills distractions, letting you excel in all pursuits—fitness, business, personal goals.
4. **Improved Self-Confidence**
   A winning mindset adds conviction to your moves, inviting respect and leadership potential.
5. **Steady Personal Growth**
   A champion's outlook emphasises continuous skill and character development.
6. **Better Emotional Control**
   Champions don't let fleeting emotions derail their path. Daily mental drills build calm under pressure.
7. **Leadership & Influence**
   Others see your unwavering determination, fueling their own drive. You become a role model.
8. **Enhanced Problem-Solving**
   Challenges become puzzles to solve, not barriers that halt progress.

9. **Stronger Connections**
Positive energy often cultivates supportive relationships with friends, family, and colleagues.
10. **Long-Term Legacy**
Sustain champion-level thinking for months on end, and you'll form habits that outlast any single project or challenge.

Consequences of Not Thinking Like a Champion

1. **Frequent Doubts & Self-Limiting Beliefs**
Without mental discipline, fear dominates, leading to hesitation or abandoned goals.
2. **Lower Resilience**
Minor setbacks might feel catastrophic, undermining your faith in your abilities.
3. **Scattered Focus & Mediocre Results**
You'll be more prone to distractions, stalling progress in key areas.
4. **Missed Opportunities**
A passive mindset often overlooks big chances to shine or level up.
5. **Weakened Emotional Control**
Stress, anger, or anxiety can derail plans when you lack champion-level mental strategies.
6. **Strained Relationships**
Negative attitudes or a defeatist mindset can affect the morale of those around you.
7. **Unfulfilled Potential**
With no champion's drive, you risk settling for comfort, never pushing your boundaries.
8. **Greater Susceptibility to Negativity**
Without mental defenses, negativity can infiltrate, hampering creativity and ambition.

9. **Inconsistent Leadership**
People may sense you waver under adversity, questioning your reliability.
10. **Long-Term Regret**
Down the line, you might wish you'd harnessed that winning mindset to create a bolder legacy.

Ali once said, "If my mind can conceive it, and my heart can believe it—then I can achieve it." Let that become your guiding principle.

Activities: Designing a Champion's Daily Mental Workout
Now that we have clarity on why we want to think like a champion, it's time to define the practical steps. Remember, we also integrate a day that "will consist of a 5km+ run and a boxing session with bagwork, shadowboxing, padwork, jump rope, floor work, stretching, etc." But the mental side is equally pivotal.

Daily Practices (20 Minutes Minimum)

1. **Affirmations & Visualisation**

    - **Morning Routine:** Upon waking, spend 5 minutes reciting power statements like "Train like a fighter" "Think like a champion," "I move with confidence.". Say your top ten goals out loud and read the 12 key principles of success affirmations.
    - **Visualisation:** Picture yourself succeeding—stepping into a ring or delivering a winning viral piece of content that inspires high achievers to box at get fit. See yourself winning the day before you have stepped out the door. Plan for success in your mind.

2. **Goal Setting & Review**

    ○ **Morning & Evening:** Jot down top objectives for the day, and in the evening, reflect on progress. Like Floyd Mayweather meticulously analysing each training session, you'll note what went well and where to improve.

3. **Mindset Work During Running**

    ○ **5 km+ Run:** Use the run to mentally rehearse your next big goal or practice mantras. Many great fighters often prayed or thought through tactics during his early runs, integrating mind and body.

4. **Spiritual or Reflective Reading**

    ○ 5-10 minutes daily of reading inspirational material—could be quotes from Ali or a short passage from a leadership book. In this case it will be the Bible. Keep your mind fed with uplifting perspectives.

5. **Boxing Session Integration**

    ○ As you do bagwork or shadowboxing, deliberately remind yourself of champion traits—persistence, confidence, skill. This transforms mere physical effort into a mental fortification exercise.

Weekly & Monthly Adjustments

- **Weekly Reflection:** Did you remain consistent with affirmations? Did you skip days? Fix that.
- **Monthly Skill-Focus:** Each month, target a mental skill—for instance, emotional control in high-stress scenarios or reframing self-talk when you catch negativity creeping in.

Quarterly Break

- After three months, give yourself a week off from structured mental training—but not from positivity altogether. Let your mind rest from the routine, or try lighter exercises like journaling your gratitude. This break helps avoid mental fatigue.

Leverage: People, Resources, and Communities to Fuel Your Mindset

You're not meant to walk this road alone. Champions often cite mentors, coaches, or communities that keep them on their toes.

People

1. **Jonathan Reid (Accountability Partner)**

    - Set up a system for him to check whether you did your 20 minutes daily. A quick text or call is enough.

2. **Tony Robbins & Other Mental Coaching Experts**

    - Absorb their strategies on peak mental performance, using personal development talks or courses to refine your champion mindset.

Resources

1. **Guided Mindset Videos on YouTube**

    - Channels dedicated to mental toughness, champion habits, or sports psychology.

2. **A Personal Book of Affirmations**
   - Craft your own and use a journal that you can update with champion-worthy statements daily.

Community

1. **David Lloyd Gym & Key Results Club**
   - Surround yourself with individuals also pursuing big goals. Shared ambition fosters synergy.
2. **The Tab Church or Spiritual Fellowship**
   - If faith is central, aligning your mindset with spiritual principles can intensify purpose and moral grounding.

"Tough times don't last; tough people do," said Floyd Mayweather Jr. Tapping into mentors, resources, and supportive groups transforms fleeting ambition into a robust fortress of positivity.

Score: Measuring "Think Like a Champion" Over 300 Days

A champion meticulously reviews each fight, or each training block. You'll do something similar to ensure you're truly building that unstoppable mentality.

Lead KPIs

1. **Daily Minutes Logged:** A simple tally—did you do your 20 minutes? 0 or 1 for each day.
2. **Morning & Evening Practice Rate:** Did you set goals in the morning and reflect at night?

3. **Affirmations/Visualisation Completion:** Quick check—did you speak or mentally rehearse your champion statements?

Lag KPIs

1. **30, 100, 150, 200, 300-Day Completion:** Each milestone marks deeper ingraining of champion-level thinking.
2. **Emotional Control & Confidence:** Harder to measure, but can you see improvements in stressful scenarios? Are colleagues or family noting your calmer demeanor?
3. **Performance Gains in Physical Training:** Does your consistent mental edge translate into faster runs, better padwork, or more consistent boxing techniques?

Celebrating Wins

- **Mini Rewards:** At 30 days, treat yourself to a new mindset or motivational audiobook. At 100 days in, maybe a short weekend getaway. At 300 days, something bigger—a personal retreat or a donation in honor of your transformation.
- **Mentor or Coach Feedback:** Periodically share your experiences with a mindset coach or accountability partner to glean external perspective on your progress.

Personal Stories & Champion Quotes

I recall a phase when I was overwhelmed juggling a new business venture, a demanding training schedule, and personal obligations. I teetered on the brink of burnout— until I decided to invest just 15 minutes each morning in mental conditioning (affirmations, reading motivational passages, visualising the day's successes). The difference was staggering. Over time, I not only coped better with stress, but I found solutions to challenges I previously deemed insurmountable. That mental clarity was reminiscent of Roy Jones Jr.'s approach, who famously said, "If you don't think you can, you won't."

Fighters like Manny Pacquiao have often shared how their spiritual routines—prayer, reading, mental centering—melded with physical drills. Pacquiao's humility and unwavering faith carried him through countless tough fights. Similarly, Mike Tyson, for all his bravado, had an almost monastic discipline at his peak, waking early, training relentlessly, and reading about historical conquerors. These stories taught me that champion thinking isn't some intangible gift but a daily craft—a craft we can all adopt.

The 12 Key Principles of Success

"Think Like a Champion for 300 Days" seamlessly dovetails with the *12 key principles of success* we've emphasized in *A Year By Design*:

1. **Faith:** Believing in your capacity to transform daily mindset practice into unstoppable mental strength.
2. **Vision:** Keeping your eyes on the long game—300 days of mental discipline shapes who you'll be next year.
3. **Teamwork:** Leaning on accountability partners, mentors, or your spiritual community for motivation.
4. **Focus:** Consistently dedicating 20 minutes, no matter how busy the schedule.
5. **Hard Work & Dedication:** Day in, day out, champion thinking becomes non-negotiable.
6. **Discipline:** Overcoming distractions, negative self-talk, or social media pulls to maintain your mental training.
7. **Will to Win:** Embracing daily obstacles as challenges, not problems.

8. **Resilience:** Bouncing back when you miss a day or slip up. Reset and go again.
9. **Confidence:** Affirmations build a deep-rooted self-belief that transcends fleeting circumstances.
10. **Respect:** Valuing yourself, your trainers, your circle. Champions don't exist in a vacuum.
11. **Humility:** Knowing there's always room to learn from losses, from mentors, from daily experiences.
12. **Legacy:** The mindsets you adopt for 300 days can linger a lifetime, shaping how you approach every future challenge.

A Call to Action: 12 Minutes to Plan Your Champion Mindset

Let's convert theory into action. *Right now*, carve out 12 minutes to do the following:

1. **Determine Your Mindset Days:** Will you also aim for 300 days, or a slightly different number to suit your calendar?
2. **Plan the Daily Routine:**

   - Where do those 20 minutes go—mornings, lunchtimes, or evenings?
   - Which mental practices (affirmations, journaling, visualisation) resonate most with you?
3. **Tie It to Physical Training:**

   - Will you do your mental routine before or after a 5 km run? Combine it with shadowboxing?
4. **Identify Accountability:**

   - Who checks up on you weekly?
   - What resources or phone apps track your progress?
5. **Reward System:**

- On day 30, 100, 150, 200, and 300, how will you celebrate or reflect?

Write these points down—turn them into a short, bullet-point plan. Champions don't just dream; they design and execute.

Build the Champion Mindset That Lasts a Lifetime

In the ring, mental warfare often decides the fight even before the first punch is thrown. The boxer who steps in with unwavering conviction already has an advantage. *Thinking like a champion* for 300 days bestows that same advantage upon your everyday life, whether you're tackling a business goal, forging better relationships, or training your body to accomplish feats you never thought possible.

This chapter is an invitation to harness that ironclad mindset, to revolve your daily routine around a steadfast 20-minute practice of affirmations, visualisation, goal review, or spiritual reading. And when you blend that with your physical training—like a consistent 5 km run or boxing session—you reinforce the synergy between mind and body.

Remember what Floyd Mayweather Jr. said: "It's not bragging if you can back it up." By day 300, you won't be bragging; you'll be living proof that champion-level thinking is available to everyone willing to invest in it. You'll have an edge in every pursuit, from the boxing ring to the boardroom, from your personal wellness journey to the impact you make on your community.

So, slip on your mental gloves. Dive into those daily 20 minutes, tie them to your training sessions, and watch as your world transforms. Because once you harness a champion's mindset, you become unstoppable in whatever arena you enter. That's the real knockout victory—a disciplined, confident, resilient you, ready to seize every opportunity life throws your way.

16

Level Up Like a Boss for 300 Days

Success is a choice—a series of deliberate actions, habits, and mindset shifts that build momentum toward greatness. For the next 300 days, I'm committing to leveling up like a boss. This isn't just about working hard; it's about working smart, building systems, and mastering the art of business. Through consistency, focus, and grit, I'll turn potential into results, dreams into plans, and plans into action.

This chapter outlines the principles and steps necessary to elevate your life and business like a true boss, guided by the G.O.A.L.S. framework.

G.O.A.L.S Framework
Gratitude

Every journey starts with gratitude—it sets the foundation for success. Here's what I'm grateful for that fuels my drive to level up like a boss:

1. **Past Wins:** I've built successful assets before and seen their impact.
2. **Entrepreneurial Independence:** Since 2021, I've charted my own course as my own boss.
3. **A Passion for Business:** I genuinely love the process of creating, innovating, and scaling ventures.

4. **Inspiring Role Models:** I'm surrounded by examples of exceptional bosses whose strategies I can learn from.
5. **Consistency in Success Principles:** The patterns of success—discipline, focus, and persistence—apply universally.

Outcome Goal:

I will level up like a boss for 300 days, dedicating myself to mastering business, building assets, and achieving measurable growth. One must invest 3 hours minimum in a day to be considered leveling up like a boss.

Checkpoints:

1. **30 Days:** Establishing systems, creating initial assets, and gaining momentum.
2. **100 Days:** Refining processes and achieving initial wins.
3. **150 Days:** Scaling reach and optimizing strategies.
4. **200 Days:** Solidifying systems for maximum efficiency.
5. **300 Days:** Evaluating success, celebrating milestones, and preparing for the next level.

Top Ten Reasons to Level Up Like a Boss

1. **Mastery of My Craft:**
   Dedicating 300 days ensures I refine my skills, dominate my niche, and create unmatched value.
2. **Financial Freedom:**
   Elevating performance leads to increased opportunities, promotions, and revenue streams.
3. **Unshakable Confidence:**
   Seeing tangible progress builds self-esteem, empowering me to take on bigger challenges.

4. **Strategic Thinking:**
Leveling up sharpens decision-making, problem-solving, and goal-setting abilities.
5. **Leadership Influence:**
By consistently improving, I inspire those around me to pursue their own growth journeys.
6. **Opportunity Creation:**
Success creates opportunities not just for me, but also for my family, friends, and community.
7. **A Lasting Legacy:**
My growth sets a blueprint for future generations, proving what's possible through discipline and hard work.
8. **Resilience Under Pressure:**
Consistent effort builds mental toughness, ensuring I can navigate challenges with grace.
9. **Accelerated Personal Growth:**
Focusing on self-improvement for 300 days ensures rapid mental, emotional, and physical development.
10. **Fulfillment Through Progress:**
The joy of reaching milestones and seeing dreams materialise fuels my sense of purpose.

What Happens If I Don't Level Up Like a Boss

1. **Career and Personal Stagnation:**
Without focused effort, I risk remaining in the same place, missing out on opportunities for growth and achievement.
2. **Regret Over Wasted Potential:**
Failing to act on my abilities will lead to frustration and disappointment in myself.

3. **Weakened Confidence:**
   Lack of progress breeds self-doubt, limiting my willingness to take on future challenges.
4. **Loss of Influence:**
   If I fail to grow, I can't inspire or lead others, diminishing my impact on my community and network.
5. **Missed Financial Rewards:**
   Growth directly correlates with financial success. Without leveling up, I'll miss the chance to provide for my family, invest in my future, and pursue my dreams.
6. **Unrealised Opportunities:**
   The doors opened by consistent success—networking, collaborations, and life experiences—will remain closed.
7. **Lower Emotional Resilience:**
   Without the discipline and focus of leveling up, I'll struggle more with setbacks and challenges.
8. **Strained Relationships:**
   Failing to grow and contribute to those around me can lead to disconnection and disappointment.
9. **Wasted Time:**
   Time is finite. Without a clear plan for growth, I risk squandering it on unproductive habits.
10. **Limited Legacy:**
    If I don't act now, I risk leaving little behind to inspire or guide future generations.

Activities

To level up like a boss, I've broken the journey into four key activities:

1. **Build Assets:**

- Create five pieces of content daily: books, blog posts, content

2. **Optimise Funnels:**

    - Generate twenty five leads daily through email marketing, landing pages, and social media campaigns.

3. **Schedule Contacts:**

    - Book five calls daily to nurture relationships and close deals.

4. **Secure Unique Partnerships:**

    - Build three meaningful collaborations daily to expand my reach and impact.

Weekly Schedule:

- **Monday:** 12–6 pm
- **Tuesday:** 11–5 pm
- **Wednesday:** 11 am–12 pm, 2–5 pm
- **Thursday:** 1–5:30 pm
- **Friday:** 11 am–6 pm
- **Saturday:** 11 am–5 pm
- **Sunday:** 3–5 pm (planning and review)

Leverage

1. **People:**

    - Jonathan Reid for accountability and systems
    - Alex Hormozi and Russell Brunson for strategies

- Tony Robbins, Bedros Keullian and Eric Thomas for mindset

2. **Resources:**

    - Books and guides on asset creation and funnel optimisation
    - Tools like ClickFunnels, lead magnets, and email automation

3. **Community:**

    - Key Results Club, business masterminds, and supportive networks

Score

I'll track progress with the following KPIs:

- **Lead Metrics:** Assets created, leads generated, calls booked
- **Lag Metrics:** Calls delivered, clients signed, revenue generated

Call to Action

Take 12 minutes to reflect on what "leveling up like a boss" means to you. Identify your key activities, sources of leverage, and progress metrics. Commit to the number of days you'll dedicate to this goal and create a plan to celebrate each milestone along the way.

Final Thoughts

To level up like a boss is to commit to your growth, lead by example, and create a legacy of excellence. Over the next 300 days, I'll push boundaries, break through barriers, and inspire others to do the same. Will you join me on this journey? Let's rise together.

17

Study Champions From The Bible

"Success is not just a result of hard work but of faith, vision, and wisdom—qualities we can learn from the great champions of the Bible."

This chapter is a deep dive into why studying biblical champions like Jesus, Moses, David, Solomon, and Samson is not just a spiritual exercise but a transformative journey. By understanding their lives, challenges, and victories, you can draw wisdom, strength, and guidance to elevate your own path. This is about growing spiritually and applying those lessons practically in every area of life.

The G.O.A.L.S Framework
Gratitude

Gratitude fuels spiritual growth by grounding us in the blessings we already have. Here's what I'm grateful for as I embark on this journey to study biblical champions:

1. **Access to the Bible:** I have the wisdom of the Bible readily available, a guidebook filled with lessons for life.
2. **Love for Learning:** I genuinely enjoy exploring biblical teachings and connecting them to my everyday life.
3. **Faith as a Foundation:** My belief in God provides clarity and direction in my actions and decisions.

4. **Examples of Great Champions:** Figures like Jesus, David, and Moses serve as timeless inspirations.
5. **A Supportive Community:** My church and spiritual leaders are always there to guide and encourage me.

Outcome
Goal:
To dedicate 20 hours of study, prayer, and fellowship to learning about five great biblical champions: Jesus, Moses, David, Solomon, and Samson.
SMART Breakdown:

- **Specific:** Study the lives and lessons of five champions from the Bible.
- **Measurable:** Invest 20 hours, broken down into daily and weekly sessions.
- **Achievable:** Use Bible readings, documentaries, and fellowship sessions to dive deeper into their stories.
- **Relevant:** Strengthen spiritual growth to align with my personal and professional goals.
- **Time-Bound:** Complete this study over the course of 50 weeks. 10 weeks per Champion.

Checkpoints:

1. Study Moses and his leadership journey.
2. Reflect on David's courage and emotional resilience.
3. Explore Solomon's wisdom and decision-making.
4. Examine Samson's strength and vulnerabilities.
5. Meditate on Jesus' teachings and ultimate sacrifice.

Top Ten Reasons to Study Champions from the Bible

1. **Timeless Leadership Lessons:**
   Moses' perseverance, David's courage, and Jesus' humility offer lessons on how to lead with strength, vision, and grace.
2. **Faith in Action:**
   These champions demonstrate unwavering faith during trials, teaching us resilience and trust in divine guidance.
3. **Decision-Making Clarity:**
   Solomon's wisdom highlights the power of discernment in making choices that align with purpose and values.
4. **Strength and Humility:**
   Samson's physical power and Jesus' compassionate humility remind us to balance strength with kindness.
5. **Emotional Resilience:**
   David's ability to overcome betrayal and loss provides a blueprint for navigating personal and professional setbacks.
6. **The Power of Vision:**
   Moses' dedication to leading his people to the Promised Land teaches us the importance of long-term goals and persistence.
7. **Sacrifice and Service:**
   Jesus' ultimate sacrifice inspires us to live selflessly and prioritize the well-being of others.
8. **Confidence in Challenges:**
   David's confidence in facing Goliath demonstrates how preparation and faith can conquer even the most intimidating obstacles.
9. **Legacy of Wisdom and Faith:**
   Solomon's teachings leave a legacy of wisdom that can guide generations to come.
10. **Deeper Spiritual Connection:**
    Studying these champions strengthens our relationship with God and gives us tools to navigate life with faith and purpose.

What Happens If You Do Not Study Champions from the Bible

1. **Lack of Perspective in Challenges:**
   Without David or Moses' examples, you may feel overwhelmed when faced with adversity, missing the faith-driven strategies they employed.
2. **Missed Wisdom for Life:**
   Ignoring Solomon's teachings could result in shortsighted decisions that lack depth or foresight.
3. **Weak Spiritual Foundation:**
   Without learning from Jesus' life, you risk losing a connection to your faith, leaving you directionless in times of uncertainty.
4. **Imbalance in Strength and Humility:**
   Neglecting Samson's and Jesus' stories may lead to an inability to balance assertiveness with compassion.
5. **Difficulty Recovering from Setbacks:**
   David's life teaches grace and recovery after failure. Without his example, you may struggle to turn failures into opportunities for growth.
6. **Limited Vision for Purpose:**
   Moses' dedication to his mission inspires us to dream bigger. Without this influence, it's easier to settle for less.
7. **Reduced Capacity for Sacrifice and Service:**
   Jesus' teachings remind us of the joy in serving others. Without these lessons, life risks becoming overly self-centered.
8. **Low Confidence in Challenges:**
   David's faith and preparation inspire courage. Without studying his example, you may hesitate in the face of daunting tasks.
9. **Weakened Leadership Skills:**
   Moses and Jesus show us how to lead with vision and empathy.

Ignoring their lessons may hinder your ability to inspire and guide others.
10. **Missed Opportunity for a Lasting Legacy:**
Without the lessons of these champions, you miss the chance to build a purposeful, impactful legacy.

Activities

To study these champions effectively, I'll incorporate the following activities:

1. **Daily Bible Study:**

    ◦ Read specific passages about each champion's journey.
2. **Prayer and Reflection:**

    ◦ Spend time meditating on how their lessons apply to my life.
3. **Watch Documentaries or Sermons:**

    ◦ Learn through visual and auditory storytelling.
4. **Group Fellowship:**

    ◦ Engage with my community to discuss insights and applications.
5. **Weekly Recaps:**

    ◦ Write a summary of key takeaways to internalise lessons.

Weekly Schedule:

- **Sunday:** Attend church and fellowship.

- **Monday to Friday:** Dedicate 30 minutes daily to Bible study and prayer.
- **Saturday:** Watch a documentary or listen to a sermon on a specific champion.

Leverage

1. **People:**

   - Pastor Mike for spiritual guidance and interpretation of lessons.
   - Accountability partners like Justina & Ope Omotayo to keep me consistent.

2. **Resources:**

   - The Bible and Bible App for reading plans.
   - Documentaries and books on the lives of biblical figures on Netflix & Prime.

3. **Community:**

   - Church groups, online Bible study communities, and fellowship events.

Score

To measure progress:

- **Lead Metrics:** Time spent in study, prayer, and fellowship.
- **Lag Metrics:** Improved spiritual understanding, actionable insights applied to daily life, and strengthened faith.

Call to Action

Take 12 minutes today to reflect on the biblical champions who inspire you. Write down three lessons you want to learn from their stories and set a plan for studying them over the next year.

Final Thoughts

Studying champions from the Bible isn't just about spiritual growth; it's about equipping yourself with timeless wisdom for life's challenges. Whether you're striving to lead, persevere, or inspire, the lessons from Jesus, Moses, David, Solomon, and Samson provide a roadmap for success. Let's journey through these stories together and emerge stronger, wiser, and more grounded in purpose.

18

Feature 12 Times in Mainstream Media

"**Visibility is the currency of influence. To inspire the world, you must be seen and heard.**"

Appearing in mainstream media is more than just a vanity metric—it's a testament to your authority, credibility, and the value of your message. It amplifies your voice and creates opportunities to impact lives at scale. This chapter is your roadmap to securing 12 mainstream media features and leveraging them to elevate your personal brand, business, and mission.

What Does It Mean to Feature in Mainstream Media?

Mainstream media refers to traditional and established outlets with broad reach, including television, radio, newspapers, and high-traffic online platforms. This can also extend to digital spaces with millions of followers, such as top-tier podcasts or YouTube channels. For this goal, "featuring" can mean being interviewed, having a story about you published, or collaborating with these platforms to share your message.

To ensure this goal is actionable, I've crafted a **SMART definition**:

- **Specific:** Secure 12 features in mainstream media.
- **Measurable:** Each feature is counted and tracked.
- **Achievable:** Leverage my existing media experience, networks, and content to pitch stories.

- **Relevant:** Align media features with my mission to inspire, motivate, and empower others.
- **Time-Bound:** Achieve 12 features by December 31, 2025.

The G.O.A.L.S Framework
Gratitude

Gratitude grounds your efforts in positivity and reminds you of the tools you already have to achieve your goal. Here are five things I'm grateful for as I pursue this milestone:

1. **Prior Media Experience:**
   My appearances on BBC Radio, *For Fitness Sake* podcast, and Kent TV have given me a strong foundation.
2. **Established Media Contacts:**
   I'm fortunate to have connections with people in media and PR, who can offer guidance and open doors.
3. **Compelling Stories to Share:**
   From boxing to business, I've accumulated experiences that resonate with diverse audiences.
4. **Access to Resources:**
   Platforms like LinkedIn, Instagram, and Eventbrite make it easier to connect with media professionals.
5. **A Mission That Matters:**
   My work as a boxing life coach, author, and entrepreneur has the potential to inspire people worldwide.

Outcome

My goal is to secure **12 mainstream media features** by the end of 2025, focusing on outlets that align with my message and audience.

SMART Breakdown:

- **Specific:** Secure 12 features across TV, radio, print, or high-traffic digital platforms.
- **Measurable:** Track each feature and its impact.
- **Achievable:** Build on my existing media experience and leverage my network.
- **Relevant:** Use media appearances to promote my books, coaching programs, and mission.
- **Time-Bound:** Complete this goal within 12 months.

Checkpoints:

1. **First Feature:** Kickstart the momentum with an impactful debut.
2. **Third Feature:** Diversify across platforms like podcasts, articles, and TV.
3. **Sixth Feature:** Midway review to assess progress and refine strategies.
4. **Ninth Feature:** Focus on high-profile opportunities.
5. **Twelfth Feature:** Celebrate the milestone with a recap of lessons learned.

Top Ten Reasons to Feature in Mainstream Media

1. **Boosted Credibility:**
   Being featured on trusted platforms solidifies your reputation as an expert in your field.
2. **Expanded Reach:**
   Mainstream outlets expose your message to thousands or even millions of new eyes and ears.

3. **Personal Brand Building:**
   Media appearances highlight your expertise and personality, creating a lasting impression.
4. **Attracts New Opportunities:**
   Media exposure can lead to collaborations, speaking engagements, and partnerships.
5. **Community Leadership:**
   Sharing your insights inspires others and establishes you as a thought leader.
6. **Increased Sales and Leads:**
   Media segments often translate into tangible business growth, from book sales to coaching sign-ups.
7. **Enhanced Influence:**
   A larger platform allows you to shape conversations and advocate for causes you care about.
8. **Motivation and Accountability:**
   Preparing for media appearances forces you to refine your message and maintain a high standard of professionalism.
9. **Global Visibility:**
   Media features can open doors to international opportunities and audiences.
10. **Legacy Building:**
    Documenting your journey through media appearances ensures your story inspires future generations.

What Happens If You Don't Feature in Mainstream Media?

1. **Limited Reach:**
   Without media exposure, your message remains confined to your existing audience.

2. **Missed Opportunities:**
Media often acts as a catalyst for new connections, collaborations, and ventures.
3. **Reduced Credibility:**
Lack of visibility might make you seem less authoritative or established in your field.
4. **Weakened Influence:**
Without a platform, it's harder to shape conversations or inspire meaningful change.
5. **Slower Growth:**
Media features drive momentum for personal and professional growth. Without them, progress may feel stagnant.

Activities

To achieve this goal, I've broken it down into daily, weekly, and monthly habits:

1. **Daily Habits:**

    - Research media outlets relevant to my niche.
    - Refine storylines that align with their audience's interests.

2. **Weekly Habits:**

    - Pitch at least three stories to media contacts.
    - Prepare for upcoming interviews or features.

3. **Monthly Habits:**

    - Secure one media feature.
    - Evaluate the impact of completed features and adjust strategies as needed.

Example Storylines:

- My journey as a boxing life coach inspiring entrepreneurs to adopt a champion mindset.
- Lessons from publishing 33 books in a year.
- How boxing principles can transform business success and personal growth.

Leverage People:

- Media professionals from DAZN, Sky Sports, iFL TV, Ring Magazine, BBC and other companies for advice and introductions.
- Mentors like Myron Golden and Gary Vaynerchuk for storytelling and branding strategies.

Resources:

- LinkedIn for outreach.
- Eventbrite for networking events.
- Content from my books and coaching programs to craft compelling pitches.
- Platforms like HARO (Help A Reporter Out) to find opportunities.

Community:

- Networks like Queensberry Promotions and Matchroom for collaborative opportunities.
- My personal and professional networks for amplification and support.

Score
KPIs:

- **Lead Metrics:** Number of pitches sent, media contacts reached, and interviews scheduled.
- **Lag Metrics:** Media features secured, audience reach, and resultant business leads.

Celebration:
Each feature is a win. Celebrate milestones by reflecting on lessons learned and sharing your success with your community.

Call to Action
Take 12 minutes today to:

1. List three media outlets you'd like to feature in.
2. Write down one story idea that aligns with their audience.
3. Research the best way to contact them.

Final Thoughts
Securing 12 media features isn't just about visibility—it's about using your platform to inspire, educate, and lead. Every interview, article, or TV segment is an opportunity to connect with people, share your expertise, and leave a lasting legacy. So, let's make headlines together—headlines that matter.

19

Planners vs Trackers

Planners and trackers are the dynamic duo of success. A planner is your roadmap, helping you outline where you want to go and how to get there. A tracker ensures you're staying on course, providing the necessary feedback to adjust and improve. Together, they create a cycle of intention, action, and progress that turns goals into reality.

Detailed Goal Planner and Goal Tracker Templates for Your Top 10 Goals

Below is a **Goal Planner** and **Goal Tracker** for each of your top 10 goals, designed to align with *A Year by Design*. These templates break down your ambitions into actionable steps while monitoring your progress.

1. Generate £300,000 Annual Turnover

Goal Planner

- **Annual Vision:** Achieve £300,000 turnover by leveraging book sales, Champ Camp memberships, sponsorships, and partnerships.
- **Quarterly Milestones:**
  - Q1: Publish 10 books, generate £75,000.
  - Q2: Secure 4 Elite Champions & 8 Diamond Lions, reach £150,000 turnover.
  - Q3: Expand Key Result Club membership to 1,500 participants.

- Q4: Launch a celebratory campaign to reach £300,000.

Goal Tracker

- **Monthly Progress:**
  - Books published.
  - Revenue from Key Results Club memberships.
  - Number of sponsors secured.
  - Partnerships secured.
- **Quarterly Results:**
  - Total revenue generated.
  - Milestones achieved vs. planned.

2. Publish 33 Books

Goal Planner

- **Annual Vision:** Publish 33 books by May 2025.
- **Quarterly Milestones:**
  - Q1: Publish 5 books.
  - Q2: Publish 28 books.
  - .

Goal Tracker

- **Weekly Activities:**
  - Chapters planned, resesarched, written and edited.
  - Books finalised (covers, formatting).
  - Books published.
- **Monthly Progress:**

- Number of books completed.
- Feedback received.

3. Complete 72 Days of Champ Camp

Goal Planner

- **Annual Vision:** Dedicate 72 days to intensive boxing training.
- **Quarterly Milestones:**
  - Q1: Complete 0 days.
  - Q2: Complete 18 days.
  - Q3: Complete 36 days.
  - Q4: Complete 36 days.

Goal Tracker

- **Weekly Activities:**
  - Number of training sessions completed.
  - Total hours trained.
- **Monthly Progress:**
  - Days of Champ Camp completed.
  - Progress in fitness metrics (speed, endurance, strength).

4. Make Weekly Memories with My Girlfriend

Goal Planner

- **Annual Vision:** Make meaningful memories every week with a girlfriend.
- **Weekly Activities:**
    - Plan unique memories or experiences (dinners, trips, activities).
    - Reflect on memories in a journal.
- **Quarterly Milestones:**
    - Q1: Make memories weekly
    - Q2: Explore new experiences with beautiful women.
    - Q3: Settle down and commit.
    - Q4: End the year with a special celebration.

Goal Tracker

- **Weekly Progress:**
    - Number of single women complimented
    - Number of memories made
- **Monthly Review:**
    - Total memories made.
    - Personal reflection on relationship growth.

5. Celebrate Success with Family and Friends

Goal Planner

- **Annual Vision:** Celebrate milestones and meaningful events with loved ones.
- **Quarterly Milestones:**
    - Q1: Host a family dinner.
    - Q2: Organise a friend's gathering.
    - Q3: Plan a celebratory outing.
    - Q4: Host an end-of-year event.

Goal Tracker

- **Monthly Progress:**
    - Number of celebrations or gatherings attended/hosted.
    - Moments shared and memories created.
- **Quarterly Review:**
    - Feedback from family and friends on connection quality.

6. Train Like a Fighter for 300 Days

Goal Planner

- **Annual Vision:** Dedicate 300 days to a fighter's training routine.
- **Quarterly Milestones:**
  - Q1: Complete 60 days.
  - Q2: Complete 75 days.
  - Q3: Complete 90 days.
  - Q4: Complete 75 days.

Goal Tracker

- **Weekly Activities:**
  - Runs completed (5km+).
  - Boxing rounds completed (bag work, sparring).
- **Monthly Progress:**
  - Total training days completed.
  - Improvements in fitness metrics.

7. Think Like a Champion for 300 Days

Goal Planner

- **Annual Vision:** Commit to champion-level thinking for 300 days.
- **Weekly Activities:**
    - Daily affirmations and visualisations.
    - Goal-setting and reflection sessions.
- **Quarterly Milestones:**
    - Q1: Build a morning mindset routine.
    - Q2: Develop emotional resilience.
    - Q3: Focus on mental clarity.
    - Q4: Celebrate mindset growth.

Goal Tracker

- **Daily Progress:**
    - Minutes spent on mindset activities.
    - Reflection on champion-level thinking.
- **Monthly Review:**
    - Total mindset days completed.
    - Improvements in focus and resilience.

8. Level Up Like a Boss for 300 Days

Goal Planner

- **Annual Vision:** Level up in business leadership and personal growth.
- **Quarterly Milestones:**
    - Q1: Build assets (books, videos, blogs).
    - Q2: Optimise sales funnels for Key Results Club.
    - Q3: Secure 10 unique partnerships.
    - Q4: Generate £300,000 turnover.

Goal Tracker

- **Weekly Activities:**
    - Assets created.
    - Calls booked
    - Unique partnerships secured
- **Monthly Progress:**
    - Revenue milestones hit.
    - New opportunities secured.

9. Study Biblical Champions
Goal Planner

- **Annual Vision:** Dedicate time to studying Jesus, Moses, David, Solomon, and Samson.
- **Quarterly Milestones:**
    - Q1: Study Moses and David.
    - Q2: Study Solomon.
    - Q3: Study Samson.
    - Q4: Study Jesus.

Goal Tracker

- **Weekly Activities:**
    - Chapters or verses studied.
    - Key lessons learned.
- **Monthly Progress:**
    - Hours spent in study and reflection.
    - Insights applied to daily life.

10. Feature in Mainstream Media 12 Times

Goal Planner

- **Annual Vision:** Secure 12 features across radio, TV, and print.
- **Quarterly Milestones:**
  - Q1: List media platforms I'd like to feature in.
  - Q2: Reach 6 features.
  - Q3: Achieve 9 features.
  - Q4: Celebrate 12 features.

Goal Tracker

- **Monthly Progress:**
  - Media contacts reached.
  - Interviews conducted.
  - Features published.
- **Quarterly Review:**
  - Total features achieved.
  - Feedback from media partners.

Call to Action

Now it's your turn. Spend 12 minutes creating a goal planner and tracker for your top ambitions. Break your vision into actionable steps, track your progress diligently, and adjust along the way. Success is built on systems—start yours today.

Please find below some planners and trackers you can use to start creating your year by design.

GOAL PLANNER 1

Goal Planner

Overall Goal		
	Outcome	Activities
Q1		
Q2		
Q3		
Q4		

INSPIRE
MOTIVATE
EMPOWER

Fight For Success

GOAL PLANNER 2

Annual Planner

Month	Goal	Activity Planner
Jan		
Feb		
March		
April		
May		
June		
July		
August		
Sep		
Oct		
Nov		
Dec		

INSPIRE
MOTIVATE
EMPOWER

Fight For Success

GOAL PLANNER 3

Monthly Planner

Overall Goal		
Week	Outcome	Activity Planner
Week 1		
Week 2		
Week 3		
Week 4		

INSPIRE
MOTIVATE
EMPOWER

Fight For Success

GOAL PLANNER 4

Weekly Time Planner

Day	Outcome	Activity Planner
Monday		
Tuesday		
Wednesday		
Thursday		
Friday		
Saturday		
Sunday		

Fight For Success

GOAL PLANNER 5

Daily Time Planner

Time	Activity Planner	Time	Activity Planner
0600		1400	
0700		1500	
0800		1600	
0900		1700	
1000		1800	
1100		1900	
1200		2000	
1300		2100	

Fight For Success

GOAL TRACKER 1

Goal Tracker

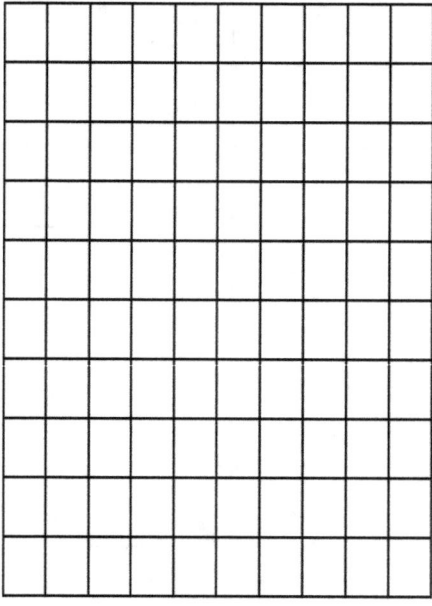

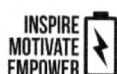

Fight For Success

GOAL TRACKER 2

Goal Tracker

Overall Goal		
	Plan	Activity Tracker
Q1		
Q2		
Q3		
Q4		

INSPIRE
MOTIVATE
EMPOWER

Fight For Success

GOAL TRACKER 3

Annual Tracker

Month	Plan	Activities
Jan		
Feb		
March		
April		
May		
June		
July		
August		
Sep		
Oct		
Nov		
Dec		

INSPIRE MOTIVATE EMPOWER

Fight For Success

GOAL TRACKER 4

Monthly Tracker

Overall Goal		
Week	Plan	Activity Tracker
Week 1		
Week 2		
Week 3		
Week 4		

INSPIRE
MOTIVATE
EMPOWER

Fight For Success

GOAL TRACKER 5

Weekly Time Tracker

Day	Plan	Activity Tracker
Monday		
Tuesday		
Wednesday		
Thursday		
Friday		
Saturday		
Sunday		

Fight For Success

GOAL TRACKER 6

Daily Time Tracker

Time	Activity Tracker	Time	Activity Tracker
0600		1400	
0700		1500	
0800		1600	
0900		1700	
1000		1800	
1100		1900	
1200		2000	
1300		2100	

Fight For Success

20

Recommended Resources

We have come to the end of the book now and it is time to live a year by design. This is not just a book to read. Follow the steps and guidance found in this book to start turning more of your goals to reality.

Please see below, some recommended reading books, along with further information about my key sponsor KELF Civil. Every winner was once a beginner, let's start working towards turning your goals into reality. Let's live a year by design and fight for success, beyond the foundation.

Reading List

1. 12 Boxing Principles of Success: Train Like a Fighter, Think Like a Champion by Kieran Ekeledo
2. Awaken the Giant Within by Tony Robbins
3. Think and Grow Rich by Napoleon Hill
4. Can't Hurt Me by David Goggins
5. Atomic Habits by James Clear
6. Your Best Year Yet by Jinny Ditzler
7. 12 Week Year by Brian Moran
8. Relentless by Tim Grover
9. How to Win Friends and Influence People by Dale Carnegie
10. Exactly What to Say by Phil M Jones
11. Shoe Dog by Phil Jones
12. Greatest ever boxing workouts by Gary Todd

KELF CIVIL

Fight For Success

- RECOMMENDED RESOURCES

LIVE A YEAR BY DESIGN

Fight For Success

LIVE A YEAR BY DESIGN

Turning dreams into reality takes more than just ambition—it requires focus, discipline, and a strategic plan. In A Year by Design, Kieran Ekeledo, the Boxing Life Coach, delivers a powerful, step-by-step guide to help business owners, aspiring entrepreneurs, and high achievers transform their biggest goals into tangible results.

Drawing from his personal journey to create his best year in 2025, Kieran shares transparent insights and actionable strategies inspired by his reflections on success, failure, and growth from 2024. This book isn't just about setting goals; it's about living with intention and crafting a future where you thrive in every area of life.

Packed with practical advice, inspirational stories, and a clear blueprint for success, A Year by Design empowers readers to:
- Clarify their vision for a purpose-driven life.
- Turn ambitious goals into actionable plans.
- Develop the mindset and habits of a champion.
- Balance personal and professional success without burnout.

Whether you're scaling your business, leveling up your fitness, or striving for meaningful personal growth, A Year by Design will equip you with the tools to make 2025 your best year yet.

If you're ready to think like a champion, act like a boss, and design a life worth celebrating, this book is your blueprint for success. Your best life starts now—let's design it together.

www.ingramcontent.com/pod-product-compliance
Lightning Source LLC
Chambersburg PA
CBHW070757020526
44118CB00036B/1877